# Sirtfood D...

*The Beginner's Cookbook Guide to Revolutionary Dieting to Activate Your Skinny Gene and Trigger Your Metabolic Energy Levels for Life: 150+ Delicious and Healthy Sirtfood Diet Recipes*

Elizabeth Lopez

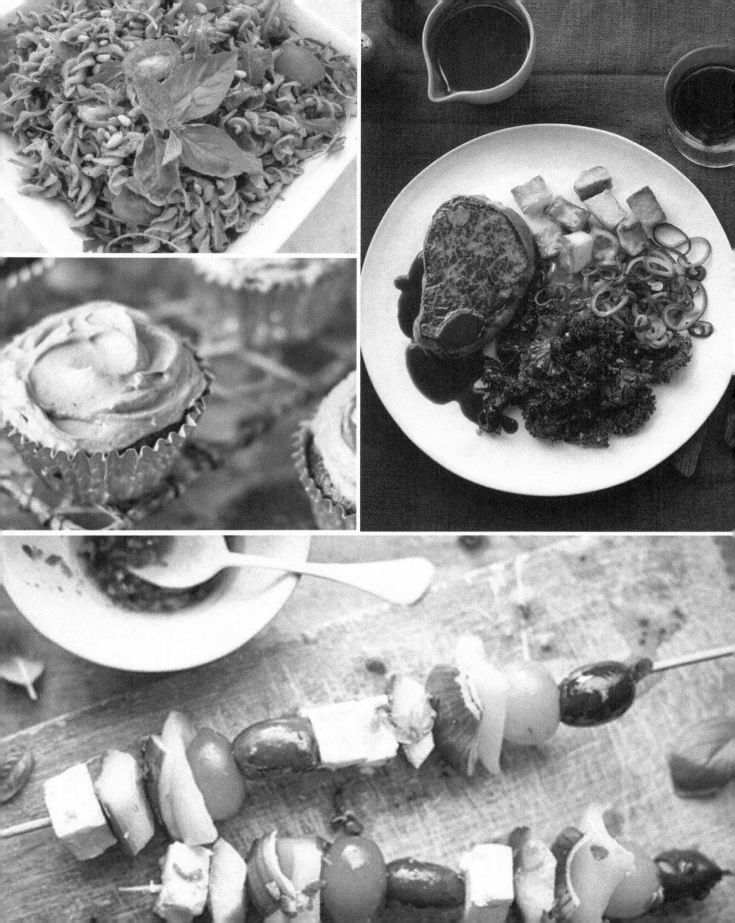

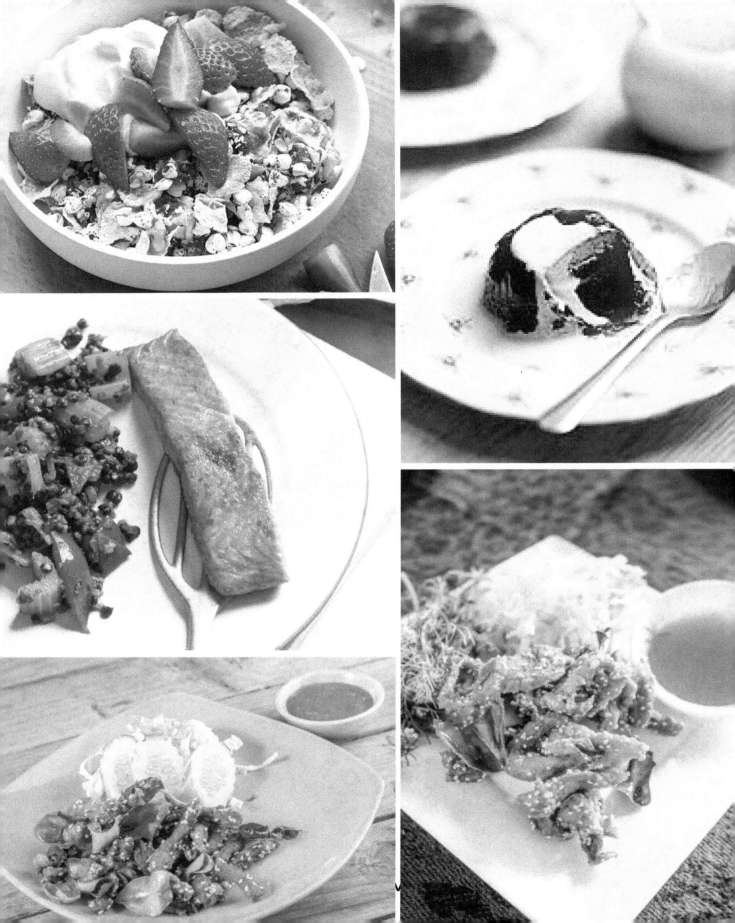

# CONTENTS

I would like to thank you for buying my book, I appreciate that. By the way, I would like to invite you to my Facebook group, where great gifts and news waiting for you. Go get Yours!

https://www.facebook.com/groups/elizabethlopezgroup

# INTRODUCTION

If I had a dollar for each time, I have come across a new diet program on the internet, I wouldn't have to work another day in my life.

There are just too many diet programme in the world today. From Keto to Paleo, from Intermittent fasting to the Mediterranean diet, from Dukan to Atkins... I could go on for hours.

Someone experimental may even combine two programme at the same time and form a new diet plan out of it. Someone could mix and match the Keto Diet with Intermittent fasting and the next thing we know, Keto Intermittent Fasting becomes a new trend.

All of these can make dieting overwhelming for people who are trying to find the perfect program to lose weight in a healthy and consistent way.

And that's not the only problem.

Most of the diet programmes out there are neither easy to do nor healthy to follow in the long run.

Many of them are based on restricting major food categories. The Keto diet, for instance, will require that you drastically limit your carbohydrate intake so that your body switches to burning stored up fat (through the so-called ketones) for energy instead of glucose.

Intermittent fasting has you starve for several hours in a day so your body can burn excess fat.

And yes, they all work. You will lose weight, but can you really eat like that for the rest of your life? The answer is no.

Therefore, it's just a waste of time because as soon as you get back to your regular eating patterns and habits you will gain all of that weight back. Sometimes with some extra pounds, which leave you worse than when you started.

A diet program will only give you permanent results when it can help you change your lifestyle and feeding patterns permanently. If you are only going to be able to do it for 2 weeks or 3 months, and then go back to eating the regular way again, I can very much guarantee that you'll gain all of the weight you lost back.

I have seen it happen so many times.

It also explains why many people are stuck in the dieting vortex for a very long time, if not for the rest of their lives.

They hear about a diet program, jump on the trend, lose some weight, go back to eating normally, or they stay disciplined and maintain their weight for a bit, then fall off the wagon at some point and start searching for the latest diet. They jump on the trend again, and the cycle continues.

Also, because most of these diets involve restricting major classes of food (e.g. low carb, low fat, etc.), they pose a potential risk to your overall health and wellbeing.

Every class of food (macronutrient) is important to your body, and vital for proper functioning of your organs. So, when you cut out major food groups, especially over a long period of time, you're depriving your body of some of the essential nutrients that it needs. It is for this reason that doctor's and dieticians often frown at most diet prog.

However, losing excess weight is important.  It is especially important if you are obese, since it may jeopardize your health sooner or later.

But regardless, you cannot sacrifice your overall health and wellbeing on the altar of weight loss - it's just not worth it. Weight loss is not worth it if it is done in a potentially harmful way.

## Why the Sirtuin diet is different

The 'Sirtuin Diet' cannot really be classified as a diet because it doesn't involve cutting out any food groups or adhering to a strict meal plan like other diet prog.

The Sirtuin Diet is different from every other diet out there because, rather than exclusion and restriction, it preaches inclusion.

Instead of cutting out foods that your body needs, or foods that your tongue craves, you include more of foods that can help you achieve speedy weight loss while still being able to eat a regular diet.

You fill up your plate with foods that can help to 'hack your skinny gene' and force your body to let go of the excess fat. And, you still get to eat the foods you love - chocolate, pasta, pizza- you name it.

The Sirtuin Diet involves cooking your meals with a lot of so-called Sirtfoods, which are the foods that can activate Sirtuins, a special group of proteins in your body.

Sirtuins help to activate your "skinny genes" and turn your body into a fat burning furnace.

You don't restrict any foods - you just add more Sirtfoods to your daily diet to achieve your final goal: weight loss.

If you think it's too good to be true, look at celebrities, like Adele, who had struggled with weight loss for years and yet managed to drop those excess pounds.

The Sirtfood Diet truly works but for it to work effectively for you, you have to do it the right way.

In this comprehensive guide, you'll find everything you need to know about this revolutionary diet.

# THE UNDERLYING POWER OF SIRTUINS FOR WEIGHT LOSS

## What are Sirtuins?

There are at least 60,000 different protein molecules in the human body and Sirtuins belong to one of those groups.

Sirtuins are a group of seven protein molecules named SIRT 1, SIRT 2, all the way to SIRT 7.

Now, to understand how Sirtuins work and how important they are, you have to picture your body as a large office where there are different departments and employees working on diverse tasks.

At the end of the day everyone has a common goal, which is to drive the success and growth of the business.

Similarly, there are different cells and organs in your body, and they are all working together towards a common goal, and that is to see that your body is healthy and functioning properly.

In a typical business organization, there is someone, or a group of people, at the helm of affairs. They make the decisions. They decide what the company's goals are, how tasks should be scheduled, and if there is a need to cut costs or change business strategies.

In your office, that is the management but at the body cellular level, the Sirtuins are the ones in charge. They are the bosses.

Sirtuins regulate cellular homeostasis, meaning that they help to maintain balance within the body, and ensure that everything is working as it should. They ensure your temperature is not too high, your immune system is not overloaded with toxins, your digestive organs are working perfectly, etc.

So, basically, they help to ensure that your body stays healthy always. In addition to this, they also protect your body cells from aging.

## SIRT 1 and Weight Loss

Of all 7 Sirtuins, SIRT 1 is the one that controls weight loss. SIRT 1 controls metabolic rate, so when you activate SIRT 1 in your body, it starts making your body switch from using glucose as energy to using fat.

Basically, it forces your body to stop storing fats and start using them.

Dr. Kushal Banerjee of the Harvard Medical School, when trying to explain how Sirtuins and SIRT 1 works for weight loss, said «SIRT 1 speeds up the metabolic rate and, therefore, the rate at which your food is burnt».

Another expert, Qiang Tong of the Baylor College of Medicine in Texas, explains the Sirtuins' effects on brown fat, that is the 'good' type of fat that keeps us warm and which we burn when we're cold (white fat is a storage depot, aka love handles): *«Obese people tend to have less brown fat than leaner people. The thinking is that Sirtuins can help activate more brown fat and help keep people lean»* - a theory that has actually been confirmed by a study published in 2012.

## Activating the Skinny Gene

We all know that one person who eats everything they want, has never had to go on a diet not even for a day, never even exercises, and still, they never gain weight.

I know a couple of people who spend lots of money on supplements that are supposed to help them gain weight. The supplements work sometimes but one stressful week, and all of the weight gain is gone.

You look at people like that and can't help but think *"Boy oh boy, this weight loss thing is rigged"* because there you are barely eating 800 calories a day, slaving it out at the gym, and you still can't lose more than a measly 2 pounds a month.

What such people enjoy is a fast metabolism. Their bodies are set up in a way that it burns fat more than it stores it.

So, when they eat, their bodies quickly go to work, using up the calories from the food to supply their bodies with energy to function. Therefore, at the end of the day, there is little to no calories left to store as fat.

On the other hand, people who gain weight easily and find it hard to lose weight often have very slow metabolism.

Their bodies are slow to utilize the energy/calories from the food they eat and end up storing most of the calories as fat. In some cases, the problem is that people actually eat more calories than their bodies need for energy, so the excess ends up being stored as fat.

This is why it is often recommended that people who are looking to lose weight should cut back on the calories they consume daily in order to create a caloric deficit. When your body cannot access all of the calories it needs to function, it will have no choice but to go into your body's fat storage and burn some of the stored fats for energy.

This simple process is what the creators of the Sirtfood Diet call 'Activating the Skinny Gene'.

Activating your skinny gene means changing the way your body uses calories and stores fat. So, your body goes from a state of excessive fat storage to extreme fat burning.

## The Problem with Calorie Restriction and Fasting for Weight Loss

But the problem with calorie restriction as a way to activate your skinny gene is that it often brings a number of challenges that make it counterproductive.

Restricting calorie consumption can cause reduction in energy levels, increased fatigue, hunger, irritability, and muscle loss.

And what most people don't realize is that the human body is very smart. We often think that we control our bodies, but the reverse is the case - our bodies control us.

The moment you start restricting the volume of food and calories your body is already used to, it gets the message that you are trying to deprive it of energy so it swings into survival mode and begins to reduce energy consumption as a way to protect your body against the effects of starvation.

So, there you are trying to reduce calorie consumption so you can lose weight, but your body is also reducing energy usage so at the end of the day, you don't lose much weight.

Long term calorie restriction is even worse because it can cause your metabolism to stagnate as your body switches fully to survival mode.

So, if you've always wondered why you are not losing much weight even when you are on a diet, this is one of the reasons.

But what if there was a way to force your body to burn more calories and fat without all of the attendant risks and side effects associated with calorie restrictions?

This is where Sirtfoods come in handy. Sirtfoods can help you activate your skinny genes without any of these negative effects - no caloric restriction, no starving.

## Eat Sirtfoods to Activate Your Skinny Genes

The relationship between Sirtuins and weight loss was first discovered in 2003, when a group of researchers discovered a plant compound called Resveratrol found in red wine and red grapes that helps to increase the lifespan of yeasts dramatically.

Upon further investigation and tests on humans, they found that Resveratrol can help to reverse the effects of a high calorie, high sugar, and high fat diet, even without restricting the consumption of these foods.

They found that a diet rich in Resveratrol mimicked the effects of both dieting and exercise. This means that just by incorporating more Resveratrol to your diet, you can lose weight and also reverse all of the common effects of eating an unhealthy diet over the years without necessarily having to adjust your diet or feeding patterns.

It was this discovery that led them to start researching similar compounds in more plants and they found several others that had the same effect on the human body.

They discovered that these plant compounds do not necessarily cause weight loss on their own. What they do is to activate SIRT 1, the Sirtuin that promotes weight loss.

Some of these Sirtuin-activating plant compounds include:

- Curcumin
- Capsaicin
- Rutin

- Polyphenols
- Quercetin
- Kaempferol
- Gingketin
- Isogingketin
- Epigallocatechin Gallate (EGCG)
- Apigen
- Fisetin
- Luteolin
- Daidzein
- Formononetin
- Myricetin

All of these plant compounds have Sirtuin-activating properties and, when you incorporate them into your diet, they provide similar effects as resveratrol, the Sirtuin-activating compound that the researchers found in red grapes and red wine.

## What are Sirtfoods?

Sirtfoods simply refer to a group of foods that are high in Sirtuin-activating compounds. Sirtfoods are rich in chemical compounds that can help boost the activities of SIRT1 and cause you to lose weight more rapidly.

Sirtfoods do not have Sirtuins in them, they only help to boost the activities of Sirtuins. It's just like adding gasoline to a vehicle - gasoline is not the vehicle itself but the vehicle cannot run without gasoline – except you got yourself a Tesla though.

Any food that is rich in the chemical compounds listed above is basically a Sirtfood; however, 20 foods were found to have the highest concentration of these compounds and are therefore regarded as the 'Top 20 Sirtfoods'.

## Top 20 Sirtfoods

1. Birds Eye Chilies

Recently, Bird's eye chilies have become very expensive and sometimes scarce in many countries around the world.

That is because people are becoming increasingly aware of the health benefits of this fruit (*yes, it's a fruit not a vegetable*), especially for weight loss. And unlike many other chili peppers, this one is grown in very little quantities.

Bird's eye chili has superb Sirtuin-activating properties but its benefits for weight loss don't end there.

Bird's eye chilies also play a key role in enhancing body metabolism. They contain a special compound called Capsaicin that creates a hot and burning sensation when you eat them. This raises your body's temperature and, in order to regulate the temperature, your body will resort to burning more calories to create body heat.

The result of this is a faster weight loss because your body will often have to turn to the unused, stored up fat deposits to make up for the increase in calorie consumption.

Other health benefits of the Bird's eye chili for weight loss include:

- Contains Antioxidant Properties: Bird's eye chilies contain at least 4 different antioxidants, among which there are capsaicin, violaxanthin, sinaplic acid, and ferulic acid. Antioxidants also improve the body's natural metabolic processes and lead to increased weight loss.
- Reduces Blood Cholesterol: Bird's eye chilies, because they contribute to the burning of old, stored up fats in the body, help to reduce the presence of the bad cholesterol, low-density lipoprotein (LDL) in the body.
- Reduces Bloating and Flatulence: If you are looking to reduce the size of your tummy and waist line, you should consider adding more Bird's eye chilies to your diet. They help to stimulate the stomach and intestinal tracts, helping to promote digestion and excretion and the result is reduced bloating and a smaller waist line.

2. Buckwheat

Buckwheat is a crop that originated from Japan. In fact, legend has it that buckwheat was such a favorite amongst Buddhist Monks that sometimes, when they made long trips to the mountains, they would go with bags of buckwheat and cooking utensils so that they could cook some buckwheat whenever they get the chance.

There wasn't so much room for cooking so they often needed foods that could keep them nourished for a very long time after a single consumption and buckwheat was one of their favorites.

Buckwheat contains rutin, a chemical compound that has Sirtuin-activating properties.

But apart from being able to help you activate your skinny genes, buckwheat also has many other benefits for weight loss.

- Improves Digestion: Buckwheat helps to speed up weight loss by improving metabolism and digestion.
- Its high fiber content helps to increase the rate at which toxins and waste products are expelled from your digestive tracts, leading to a faster metabolism and increased weight loss.
- Reduces Blood Cholesterol: With regular consumption, buckwheat can help reduce your bad cholesterol (low-density lipoprotein (LDL) levels.
- Reduces Blood Sugar: It is often tagged as a 'diabetic friendly' food because it has a low glycemic rate, which means that its glucose is absorbed much more slowly, which helps keep your blood sugar levels balanced.
- A balanced blood sugar level plays a significant role in weight management because reduces food cravings and your overall appetite.
- Promotes Gut Flora: Buckwheat also helps to stimulate the growth of healthy bacteria in the gut, which contributes to increased food digestion and absorption, and a reduction in weight gain, especially in the stomach and waist area.

3. Medjool Dates

Medjool dates are sweet, actually extremely sweet, since they have a sugar content of about 66%. So, it's only normal that you'll be wondering what this seemingly abominable food for weight loss is doing in a weight loss diet plan.

But even though Medjool dates have a high sugar content, its high polyphenol properties make it a very great food to include in a weight loss diet because polyphenols are Sirtuin-activating.

Also, the sugar in Medjool dates is different from refined or artificial sugars, which are the ones that are often problematic.

If you have a sweet tooth, and often find it hard to do without sugars on a diet, then Medjool dates are for you. You can even have them dried and grinded, and use the powder to sweeten your teas, smoothies and cereals.

This is way healthier than using table sugar, honey, syrup, or any other sweetener with a high glycemic index.

Medjool dates also have other weight loss properties and benefits:

- Prevent and Relieve Constipation: Medjool dates have a high soluble fiber content that helps bulk up your stool and make it move through your intestines faster and more easily.

If you often suffer from constipation, especially when you are on a diet, Medjool dates are good for you.

- Boost Energy Levels: One common problem people face during a diet is low energy levels. Because you are not eating as much food as your body is used to, or because your foods now contain less sugars and artificial sweeteners, you may begin to experience lower energy levels or outright body weakness that makes it difficult for you to get through your daily activities.

Medjool dates contain healthy and natural glucose, fructose and sucrose that can easily be processed and utilized by your body for energy.

4. Rocket/Arugula

In some recipes you'll see it written as arugula and some recipes call it rocket – but it's the same thing.  It is even called rucola, roquette, or arugula in some countries.

Whatever it is called in your country, the most important thing you need to know about this leafy green is that it is rich in Quercetin and Kaempferol, two Sirtuin-activating compounds.

The Romans and Ancient Greeks used it as a digestive aid in the past.  It is also believed to have aphrodisiac properties, which led it to be banned in Monasteries during the Middle Ages.

Arugula is fantastic for helping you activate your skinny genes, but it also helps you lose weight and manage your weight in several other ways:

- Has Antioxidant Properties: Arugula contains powerful antioxidant properties that promote the removal of toxins and bad cholesterol from the body.
- Restores body pH levels: Arugula is an alkaline food, which means it helps reduce acidity in your body, and helps you maintain a balanced pH level.

What does that have to do with weight loss, right? A balanced pH can help you burn stored up fats faster and keep your body from accumulating fat.

It also helps to promote gut flora, and improve digestion, which contribute to weight loss.

- **Contains Loads of Nutrients:** Arugula supplies your body with a lot of essential vitamins, nutrients and phytonutrients.

This is great for people who are into portion control or calorie counting.

It helps you get all the essential nutrients that your body needs like Vitamin K, Calcium, Magnesium, and a load of others, without eating excessively.

- **Fights Blood Sugar Fluctuations:** Fluctuations in blood sugar levels is one of the biggest culprits of overeating, especially eating of junk or sugary foods.

Increased blood sugar levels make you crave unhealthy foods, the same way abusing drugs make you crave more drugs.

Blood sugar balancing foods like arugula helps to correct this problem by reducing sugar cravings, keeping your appetite in check, and subsequently, helping you lose weight.

## 5. Capers

You're probably already familiar with capers, especially if you are a pizza lover as they are often used as pizza toppings.

They are also often featured in the Mediterranean diet as they have their origin from the Mediterranean area, that is South Europe and North Africa.

Capers contain several Sirtuin-activating compounds like phenols, quercetin, kaempferol, gingketin, and isoginkgetin.

They also have other properties that contribute to weight loss such as:

- **Improve Fat Breakdown:** Capers help improve the breakdown of fatty cells and contribute to overall weight loss.
- **Increase Sugar Uptake:** Capers can also help slow down blood sugar fluctuations by reducing the sugar uptake in your gut.

Asides their weight loss properties, capers also have antiviral and anti-cancer properties, which make them a must-have in every diet.

## 6. Celery

Celery has been used to cleanse and detox the body for thousands of years. It was also used to heal liver, kidney, and gut health problems in the ancient times.

Recently, celery has become more popular amongst dieters. In fact, many people swear by the Celery Juice Diet, a detox program that has you drink celery juice every day for several days or weeks.

Celery is one of the top Sirtfoods and consuming it regularly poses a lot of health and weight loss benefits:

- Dissolves Fat Cells: Celery helps to dissolve fat cells, especially those ones stored in the liver, leading to improved liver function, metabolism, and overall weight loss.
- Helps with Appetite Control: When you consume celery (as veggies not as juice), it fills you up for a very long time, which leads to lesser appetite and cravings, and a reduced overall food intake.
- Reduces Cholesterol Levels: Celery can also lead to a significant reduction in overall cholesterol levels.

## 7. Cocoa

Who doesn't love a diet that allows you to have chocolate? Other diets may require that you stay far away from it, but on the Sirtfood diet you get to have as much as you want because cocoa, the major ingredient in chocolate, has Sirtuin-activating properties.

But you can't have just any chocolate you may find on the supermarket shelf. You can only have brands that contain 85% cocoa solids or more.

Brands with fewer cocoa solids have diminished Sirtuin-activating properties and cannot be classified as Sirtfoods.

Other benefits of cocoa for weight loss include:

- Promotes Sleep and Reduces Stress Levels: Stress contributes to overeating and lack of sleep contributes to weight gain.
- Cocoa helps to calm the nerves and reduces stress levels and anxiety, leading to enhanced sleep and healthier eating habits.
- Promotes Digestion and Excretion: Cocoa is also rich in fiber and flavonoids that contribute to detoxification and elimination of toxins and waste from

the body.

- Improves Metabolism: Cocoa is also a thermogenic enhancer. It helps to improve weight loss by increasing the rate at which your body utilizes calories for energy.

8. Coffee

You probably wouldn't have guessed that coffee could make it on the list of foods with 'health benefits' especially since they are often demonized because of their caffeine content.

*"Caffeine is bad for you", they say; "Choose decaffeinated beverages"*, **they advise.**

While it is true that caffeine is not good for everyone, it is not true that caffeine is dangerous or shouldn't be consumed at all.

Coffee is not just one of the most powerful Sirtfoods, it also contains chlorogenic acid, a chemical compound that helps to slow down the production of glucose in the body.

Other benefits of coffee for weight loss include:

- Reduces the Production of New Fat Cells: Coffee reduces the rate at which new fat cells are produced in your body, leading to reduced fat storage and increased fat loss.

- Has Antioxidant Properties: If you are a frequent coffee drinker, you probably already know this. Coffee speeds up digestion and excretion and increases the rate at which toxins are expelled from your body.

- Suppresses Hunger: Coffee also helps to suppress hunger. It contains chemical compounds that when absorbed in the blood stream, helps to create feelings of fullness in the gut.

- Decreases Water Weight: Coffee acts as a diuretic, which means it makes you urinate often, leading to a reduction of excess fluid retention, and water weight in your body.

Of course, like I mentioned earlier, coffee is not for everyone especially if you have underlying health issues that make coffee a health risk for you.

If you can't have caffeine, it's okay to leave coffee out of your diet – you'll still have more than a dozen other Sirtfoods to choose from.

But if you are allowed to have decaffeinated coffee, you can opt for that because decaf coffee contains peptide tyrosine tyrosine, a chemical compound that reduces hunger, and increases satiety.

## 9. Extra Virgin Olive Oil

On the Sirtfood diet, you will have to ditch all other cooking oils and start making your food exclusively with Extra Virgin Olive Oil.

Extra Virgin Olive Oil contains Sirtuin-enhancing properties, and has other benefits for weight loss including:

- Contains Oleic Acid: Olive oil has oleic acid, which helps it to retain all of its antioxidant properties.
- Enriched with Monounsaturated Fatty Acids: Unlike many other cooking oils that contain saturated fats which make them unhealthy for cooking and frying, Extra Virgin Olive oil is a healthier choice as it contains Monounsaturated Fatty Acids, which experts have labeled 'the good fat'.

## 10. Matcha Green Tea

Another super Sirtfood is Matcha green tea. Green tea, especially Matcha green tea, contains catechins, a group of powerful flavonoids that promote fat loss.

One type of catechins that is primarily found in Matcha green tea, Epigallocatechin Gallate (EGCG), is indeed a Sirtuin activator.

Matcha is processed in a particular way which makes it retain its EGCG properties, unlike other types of green tea.

Green tea also promotes weight loss and weight management due to the fact that:

- Improves Breakdown of Fat Cells: Before your body can burn down the excess fat that it has accumulated over time, it must first break down the fat cells.

Some special foods such as green tea however contribute to the breakdown of fat cells by inhibiting norepinephrine, an enzyme that often prevents easy breakdown of fat cells.

- Improves Fat Burning During Workout: If you have an active lifestyle or you work out regularly, consuming Matcha green tea will help to increase the rate at which your body burns fat during physical activities.

- Reduces Appetite: **Just like coffee, Matcha green tea suppresses your appetite and helps you make healthier food choices.**
- Helps Burn Stubborn Abdominal Fat: **We all know how tough it can be to lose belly fat, the type of fat that lodges in your stomach, but Matcha green tea has been proven to be helpful for getting rid of this type of fat.**

11. Kale

Everyone loves and eats kale, or don't we all? Well, we all should because kale is another super Sirtfood, thanks to its quercetin and kaempferol contents.

Kale is also great for weight loss because it:

- Acts as a Hunger Suppression: **A single cup of kale has around 2.4 g of dietary fiber, and as you already know by now, fiber keeps you filled up for a very long time and prevents hunger.**
- Contains Glucosinalate and Sulphur Compounds: **Kale is filled with two very strong detoxifiers – sulphur compounds and glucosinalate.**
- Both help to rid the body of toxins that make it harder for your body to break down and utilize stored up fats.
- Has Low Energy Density: **Researchers have revealed that consuming foods with low energy density like kale can help you lose weight faster.**

In one study conducted on a group of 200 obese women, the researchers found that subjects who consumed 2 servings of low energy-dense soup everyday lost 50% more weight compared to people who consumed high energy-dense foods.

In simpler words, it means that if I consume 3 meals of 250 calories each (750 calories in total), but with fewer kilocalories per gram, and you consume the same quantity of meals with similar calorie count but with a higher count of kilocalories per gram, I will most likely lose weight faster than you even though we're pretty much eating the same number of calories daily.

12. Lovage /Sea Parsley

It is important to not confuse lovage with flat-leaf parsley.

If you live in the US, you're probably more familiar with flat-leaf parsley, which is commonly used to garnish and spice up your meals.

But lovage is another member of the parsley family that is also known as sea parsley. Take note of this when you go grocery shopping so you can buy the right type of parsley.

Lovage contains apigen, another superb Sirtuin-activator. Lovage is also great for people who suffer from insomnia as apigen can bind to the benzodiazepine receptors in the human brain, helping to calm you down and promote sleep.

In addition to be a Sirtfood, lovage also helps with:

- Digestion: Lovage promotes digestion and gastrointestinal health. It also reduces stomach bloating and gastrointestinal inflammation.
- Kidney Health: A healthy functioning kidney is crucial to weight loss and weight management and lovage helps to promote kidney health by promoting detoxification and urination.

And you know what the best thing about lovage's diuretic effect is? It doesn't cause electrolytes loss like most diuretics do.

13. Red Chicory

Red chicory is a common secret ingredient in many weight loss herbal teas and supplements.

It is a Sirtuin-activator, and it also has many other weight loss benefits.

- Contains Inulin: Red chicory is made up of 68% inulin, a type of carbohydrate that acts as a prebiotic.

It feeds the good bacteria in your gut, which is very important because these good bacteria help to fight off the bad bacteria that are often responsible for inflammation and many other digestive issues.

- Improves Blood Sugar Control: Inulin also helps to improve blood sugar balance. It promotes carbohydrate absorption and helps to prevent blood sugar fluctuations.
- Regulates Appetite: A group of researchers conducted a study where they placed 48 obese adults on 21 g of red chicory-derived oligofructose daily for 12 weeks.

They discovered that that oligofructose helped to reduce ghrelin, the hormone that stimulates hunger.

The participants reported less hunger and cravings and had better control of their appetite.

14.  Red Endive

Red endives are rich in luteolin, another Sirtuin-activating compound. It helps to activate your skinny gene, and also helps with:

- Helps to Keep Energy Levels Stable: Any successful weight loss program must have this important element. It must be able to keep your energy levels balanced.

If your energy levels keep fluctuating, it is unlikely that you'll be able to follow through with the diet and red chicory really helps with balancing your energy levels.

- Slows Down Digestion: Red chicory also helps to slow down digestion, not in the way that you get constipated, but in a way that keeps you satiated for longer periods and keeps your appetite in check.
- Rich in Antioxidants: Endives are also rich in powerful chemical compounds that neutralize free radicals and prevent cell damage.

15.  Red Onions

The aromatic effect of red onions in your meals is enough reason for anyone to fall in love with them but its benefits surpass food flavoring.

Red onions are a rich source of the Sirtuin-activating compound, quercetin. In fact, of all the foods on this list, red onions have the highest amount of quercetin in them.

Other reasons why red onions are great for weight loss include:

- Powerful Probiotic Food: Red onions, just like red chicory, contribute to gut health as they help to feed the good bacteria in your gut. This helps to prevent bloating and reduce abdominal fat.
- Good Source of Fiber: Red onions are also a great source of fiber and help to reduce hunger and regulate appetite.

16.  Red Wine

Yayyy! A diet that allows you to drink alcohol, who would have thought?

The Sirtfood diet is not one of those diets that won't allow you to have alcohol. On this diet you can drink a glass of red wine daily as red wine is also Sirtuin-activating.

Women can have one 5-ounce glass of red wine, while men can have up to two 5-ounce glasses of red wine every day. You can also cook with it too.

Recommended red wine brands for the Sirtfood diet include Merlot, Pinot noir, and Cabernet Sauvignon.

17. Soy

Soy is a rich source of the Sirtuin activator, daidzein. It is also rich in another Sirtuin activator, formononetin.

However, you must avoid heavily processed soy products and opt for natural sources like tofu, miso, tempeh, and natto as the natural, unprocessed ones retain the Sirtuin-activating compounds you need.

Soy also promotes:

- Satiety: Soy is rich in proteins, and it is a well-known fact that protein is very great for suppressing your appetite.
- Appetite Control: Soy has a low glycemic index and can help with hunger prevention and appetite control.

18. Strawberries

Strawberries are great Sirtuin-activators too as they contain the plant compound, fisetin.

Strawberries also promote weight loss by:

- Boosting Metabolism: Strawberries are rich in anthocyanins, another chemical compound that promotes the production of adiponectin, a hormone that helps to speed up metabolism and weight loss.
- Helping to Reduce Fat: Strawberries are also rich in gallic acid which promotes the normal functioning of weight reducing hormones that are often blocked by chronic inflammation.

19. Turmeric

Turmeric contains curcumin. Curcumin is another Sirtuin-activating compound.

However, for your body to be able to properly and effectively absorb curcumin from turmeric, you have to combine it with black pepper, or cook it in fat or add it to a liquid or teas. This helps to promote the absorption of curcumin in your body.

Turmeric also aids:

- Prevention of Metabolic Syndrome: Metabolic syndrome is often characterized by fat accumulation around your abdomen and is caused by insulin resistance.
- Turmeric helps to prevent and control metabolic syndrome by controlling blood sugar levels, cholesterol, and triglycerides.
- Increases Bile Production: Turmeric increases production of bile in the stomach, which helps to aid food digestion.

20. Walnuts

Walnuts are often listed as one of the top nuts for weight loss and rightly so. Walnuts are Sirtuin-activating, help suppress hunger, and help with appetite control.

## Sirtfoods versus superfoods

This is a question I get all the time – aren't these just superfoods?

Well, Sirtfoods can be considered as superfoods too. If Sirtfoods and superfood were humans, we would say that they are cousins as they both have many similar properties, and both serve many similar purposes and significantly benefit the inner workings of the body.

But Sirtfoods all have weight loss and fat burning properties, along with being Sirtuin-activators.

Chia seeds, maca, and fenugreek for instance, are superfoods, but these are known for contributing to weight gain rather than weight loss.

So, Sirtfoods are not necessarily superfoods even though they may be classified as superfoods.

# WHAT IS THE SIRTFOOD DIET?

Now that you know all about Sirtuins and how they work to activate your skinny genes, understanding what the Sirtfood diet is, and how it works is very easy.

The diet simply involves incorporating the most powerful Sirtfoods into your daily diet.

The Sirtfood diet ensures that you eat the right quantity, variety, and form of Sirtfoods that are powerful enough to supercharge your Sirtuins (SIRT1) and force your body to start burning more fats instead of storing them.

The diet also blends Sirtuin-activating foods with the regular foods that you eat on a daily basis so that you don't have to wake up and change your feeding patterns drastically as that is the first step towards failure when dieting.

And with the Sirtfood diet ensures that you are still eating the foods that you are used to - pizza, ice cream, mac and cheese, etc. but in a way that it is filled with ingredients that have Sirtuin-activating properties.

## Fulfilling Your Daily Sirtfood Quota

You might be wondering, but I eat most of these so-called Sirtfoods, why haven't I lost weight? Well, it's not just about eating Sirtfoods, you have to eat enough of it to provide weight loss effects.

It is true that most people eat Sirtfoods daily but unfortunately, they don't eat them purposefully in a way that can lead to weight loss.

Let me explain: of all the Sirtuin-activating compounds listed earlier, 5 of them are considered to be the most powerful:

- Myricetin
- Quercetin
- Apigenin
- Luteolin

- Kaempferol

When researchers measured how much of the Sirtuin-activating compounds people consumed on average daily, they found that Americans only consumed around 13 mg of these compounds daily.

They also compared American intake of Sirtfoods to Japanese intake, and they discovered that the Japanese consumed 5 times more Sirtuin-activating compounds daily. I guess this explains why Japanese are usually slimmer and have fewer percentages of people struggling with weight loss.

In the Sirtfood diet trial conducted by Aidan Goggins and Glen Matten, they placed the subjects of the trial on hundreds of milligrams of Sirtfood-activating compounds daily, and it was immensely successful.

Overweight subjects began shedding excess pounds like melting ice. So, the Sirtfood diet involves eating, not just a miserly 13, 20, or even 50 milligrams of Sirtuin-activating compounds daily.

## How Much Sirtfoods do you Need to Eat Daily to Lose Weight?

Basically, you have to eat hundreds of milligrams of Sirtuin-activating compounds daily.

But because it can be very hard for a layman to determine the milligrams of Sirtuin-activating compounds in the foods they eat daily, a simple way to ensure that you're fulfilling your Sirtfood quota is to eat at least 5 different Sirtuin-activating compounds daily.

So, for instance, you already know that buckwheat has rutin, arugula has quercetin and kaempferol, and capers have quercetin, kaempferol, gingketin, and isogingketin.

So, when planning your meals daily, you must ensure that you have buckwheat, rocket, and capers. By incorporating these three meals into your diet for the day, you would have fulfilled your Sirtfood quota for the day, because you are having up to 5 Sirtuin-activating compounds (in this case, more) daily.

That's pretty much how it works so plan your meals in a way that you have at least 5 different Sirtuin-activating compounds daily.

## The Importance of Juicing on the Sirtfood Diet

Now, it can be really tough to fulfill your daily Sirtfood quota, especially if you are the busy type who hardly has time to cook their own meals.

That's where juices and smoothies come in handy.

A single glass of smoothie can be a quick way to fulfill your daily quota.

Let's say you make a glass of juice that has Medjool dates, arugula, celery, kale, and cocoa in it, you'll have fulfilled your daily quota of Sirtfoods for the day, and you wouldn't have to do a single minute of cooking.

Let's say, by lunch or dinner you have another smoothie or juice with another mix of Sirtfoods - that's like being in Sirtfood diet heaven because you would have had more than enough Sirtfoods for the day.

And then you can go ahead to eat your regular meals as though you're not on a diet.

It's really that simple.

## Basic Rules and Principles of The Sirtfood Diet

Now, a few ground rules and principles that help to ensure that you get fast and long-lasting results on the Sirtfood diet:

- Eat 5 Sirtfoods a Day: We already talked about this, but it is important to reiterate so you can always keep this in mind as one of the rules and principles of this diet.
- Drink 2 'Sirtified' Juices/Smoothies a Day: Have one glass of Sirtfood-powered juice with your lunch, and a glass of red wine with your dinner.
- You can never go wrong with this combination. It will help ensure that regardless of what you eat, you're at least fulfilling your daily Sirtfood quota.
- Eat Early: This is very important, Aiden Goggins and Glen Mattens, the creators of this diet, hammered on the importance of this in their book.

In their words, «*When it comes to eating, our plan simply is, the earlier the better. Ideally, finish eating by 7PM*».

They explain that eating early helps to activate the satiating effects of Sirtfoods. When you eat your Sirtfoods early it helps to keep you full for long periods and helps to keep your appetite in check throughout the day so as to prevent those food cravings and hunger pangs that force you to eat junk.

The other reason, they explain, is that when you eat early, and stop eating by 7 PM, it helps to calibrate your feeding habits with your internal body clock (Circadian Rhythm).

They explain that our body clock gears us up to handle foods most efficiently during the daylight hours because this is when our bodies are usually most active.

By 7 PM, your body is already slowing down, and any food you eat at this time will be slowly processed and that is one of the reasons why some people develop metabolic problems.

They backed this up with numerous studies that have been conducted on night shift workers, which have shown that on average, they suffer more from metabolic diseases due to their late eating patterns.

So, on this diet, you have to start eating early, and by 7PM daily, you should have had your last meal for the day.

- East Tasty Meals: This diet is against all forms of punishment and torture.

Any diet that has you eating bland, tasteless meals that you don't enjoy, will often lead to diet abandonment, where you basically abandon the diet halfway, and tell yourself *«Self-love is the most important thing»*, *«Love yourself the way you are»* and all those resign-to-fate phrases that you use to justify being overweight when a diet is too tough for you even though you know that weight loss isn't just about the aesthetics, and has more to do with safeguarding your health and well-being, and rid yourself of the underlying effects of being overweight.

Aiden Goggins and Glen Mattens explain that 'happy taste buds' are crucial to the success of this diet. You have to keep your taste buds happy through the seven major taste bud receptors.

This means that your meals must have elements of:

- Sweet
- Sour
- Salty
- Bitter

- Umami
- Pungent
- Astringent

Some ways to incorporate those elements into your diet include:

- Sweet: Eat strawberries and dates often.
- Sour: Eat strawberries.
- Salty: Eat fish and celery.
- Bitter: Eat kale, cocoa, green tea, Extra virgin olive oil, and endives.
- Umami: Eat fish, meat, and soy.
- Pungent: Add Extra virgin olive oil and garlic to your meals regularly.
- Astringent: Indulge in wine and green tea.

Incorporating these into your diet will stimulate your taste buds, allow you get more gratification from the foods you eat, and help to keep your appetite in check.

- Eat a Lot of Proteins: Your foods have to be a perfect blend of Sirtfoods and proteins.

Proteins are very important to this diet too because dietary proteins contain something called leucine, which helps to stimulate SIRT 1 to improve blood sugar control and burn more fat.

Leucine also helps to stimulate muscle building and energy supply.

So, don't skip out on your proteins on this diet. I've provided a lot of protein-packed recipes into this book so that you can enjoy a perfect blend of the foods you need to be having.

- Please, eat: If I could print this phrase in very large fonts on the cover of this book, I would. But we won't want a tacky cover now, would we?

Okay, what I'm saying is, it is important to eat on this diet. Please, do not combine this diet with intermittent fasting or any other restrictive diet.

Starvation diets are counterproductive - they are not sustainable and there is a high chance of gaining the weight back.

Also, it is more about the quality of your foods not the quantity. You can count calories if you want but don't be obsessed with calorie counting. Focus on food quality (Sirtfood, proteins, more whole foods, less packaged foods) and less on calorie consumption.

## Sirtfood Diet Phases

The Sirtfood diet comprises of 2 phases:

- Phase One: This is the beginning phase where you get to activate your skinny genes.

*This is the stage where you lose a whopping 7 pounds a day. But there are some rules you will have to follow.*

1. Eat 1 main meal and 3 Sirtfood green juices a day for the first 3 days.
2. Your entire food intake for the first 3 days has to be restricted to 1,000 calories daily.
3. From day 4 till day 7, eat 2 main meals and 2 Sirtfood green juices daily.
4. Your entire calorie intake from days 4 to 7 should not be more than 1,500 calories.

These are the rules you would have to follow for the first 7 days to lose your first 7 pounds.

I know you are already asking yourself why you have to count calories and endure meal restriction since I already said this diet won't have you do any of that, but the restrictions are only for the first 7 days and it is so that your body can get a total reset and your body can be rid of all of the toxin, inflammation, metabolic syndrome, insulin-resistance, and all of the other factors that have been working against your weight loss so far.

The first seven days is like an onboarding experience - it gets your body more friendly and receptive of Sirtuin activators.

This period will also help to activate SIRT 1 because you would be filling up your body with more Sirtuin-activators than anything else.

- Phase Two: This is the stage where you either continue to lose weight, or simply maintain your results from phase one if you don't want to lose more weight.

This stage should last for 14 days and you don't need to count calories at all at this stage.

Here are the rules for Phase two:

1. Eat 3 Sirtfood-rich meals comprising at least 5 Sirtuin-activating compounds daily.
2. Drink one Sirtfood-rich juice daily. Preferably as breakfast.
3. Eat 1 Sirtfood bite snack daily.
4. Eat your breakfast first thing in the morning and your dinner before 7PM daily.

If you still have more excess weight to lose after this stage, you can simply continue with this phase until you've lost all of the weight you want.

After this phase, there is an unofficial phase called the "Sirtfood for life" phase. This is not exactly a phase but a way to change your lifestyle and habits, so you never have to deal with excess weight or obesity again.

## Sirtfood for Life

This is the stage where you maintain your results and say bye bye to dieting for the rest of your life.

You simply need to incorporate all the things you have learnt on this diet into your daily life for the rest of your life.

Things like:

- Making sure all your meals for the day contain at least 5 Sirtuin-activating compounds.
- Drinking one Sirtfood-rich juice or smoothie daily
- Eating all your meals before 7PM.
- Ensuring that your food has all 7 elements that help to keep your taste buds happy.
- Eating protein-rich meals daily.

## Is the Sirtfood Diet Effective?

Yes, the Sirtfood diet is very effective. I and several of my clients have successfully lost weight on the Sirtfood diet. But don't take my word for it, let's talk about famous people whom you already know, and can look up yourself as a lot of celebrities have credited this diet for their dramatic weight loss after struggling for years.

Recently, singer Adele shocked the world when she, who used to be no less than a size 16 or 18, came out looking like a size 8. She credited the Sirtfood diet for her dramatic weight loss, and said she lost 7 stones (98 pounds/44.5 Kg on the Sirtfood diet).

Pippa Middleton came out looking very slim on her wedding day. She also credited the Sirtfood diet for helping her achieve that dramatic loss before her big day.

There are dozens of testimonies on the internet about this diet from people who have successfully lost weight with it so yes, it works.

Knowing what you know now about the weight loss powers of Sirtfoods (asides being Sirtuin-activators), I'm sure you would already understand why this diet is so effective.

# THE HEALTH BENEFITS AND SIDE EFFECTS

Yes, you would lose weight, and you would be able to fit in your skinny jeans, and your friends wouldn't be able to hid their shock and admiration when they see the new you, and maybe you would even make headlines like our dear singer Adele, but that is not where the benefits of this diet ends.

Along with weight loss and weight management, the Sirtfood diet also offers a lot of health benefits.

## The Health Benefits of the Sirtfood Diet

These are all the benefits you will enjoy following the Sirtfood diet:

- Muscle Gain: **This is everyone's dream - we all want to lose weight without losing muscle tone. We don't want the loose skin and flabby abs, stomachs, and breasts that drastic weight loss often leaves behind.**

The Sirtfood diet will help you achieve this dream because it incorporates a lot of proteins in your daily diet, which help to promote muscle gain during fat loss.

- Diabetes: If you are suffering from diabetes or already showing symptoms of pre-diabetes, this diet can help to reboot your body and stop insulin resistance, which is often a precursor to diabetes.

- Memory Improvement: **Some of the meals you'll be having on this diet, such as turmeric, are known to help with cognition problems and help with memory improvement.**

- Lowers Blood Pressure and Improves Cardiovascular Health: **By helping to rid the body of bad cholesterol and triglycerides that often block the arteries and make it harder for your body to pump blood, leading to high blood pressure.**

- Boosts Energy: **The Sirtfood diet, unlike many other diets that leave you feeling weak and under-motivated, helps to boost your energy levels** along with improving concentration so that it is easier for you to be productive, and be your usual self even though you are on a diet.

- Appetite Control: Inability to control appetite is often a clog in the wheel of progress on any weight loss diet.

Sirtuins will not only help you control your appetite by reducing blood sugar spikes, but it will also help to improve hormone balance so that your hunger and satiety hormones, ghrelin and leptin can start working normally again.

- Healthy Hair, Skin and Nails: Most of the Sirtfoods contain ingredients that help to boost hair, nail and skin health so get ready to glow and have better hair and nails on this diet.

- Boosts Fertility: This diet is also rich in vegetables, fruits and superfoods that are known to help boost fertility.

It can also help to reverse the symptoms of Polycystic Ovary Syndrome (PCOS), which is often linked to obesity and excess weight.

## The Risks and Side Effects

Personally, I didn't suffer any negative side effects on the diet, and neither did any of my clients however, the International Food Information Council Foundation outlined some of the risks and side effects of these diet, which I have a moral obligation to let you know about.

It is now up to you to decide if you still want to continue with this diet after learning about all of the risks and side effects.

- The Sirtfood Diet Measures Success Only in Terms of Weight Loss: The foundation expressed concerns about the fact that the Sirtfood diet only focuses on weight loss, explaining that weight loss is not necessarily a determinant of good health, and the Sirtfood diet ignores all of the benefits of food, and chooses to focus on weight loss alone.

My Opinion: I think the person or persons that came up with this just read a blog post that summarizes the diet and didn't really take time to understand this diet. If there is any diet that stresses the importance of food, and is health conscious, it is the Sirtfood diet.

We are taught to eat, to fall in love with food, and to avoid restriction. The only time when we have to do any restriction is in the first 7 days and I don't think that is too much sacrifice for permanent and sustainable weight loss.

- **The Sirtfood Diet is Not Backed by Science:** The foundation also raised concerns that there isn't enough scientific evidence.

**Let me quote them directly. On their website they wrote:** *«While there is some controversial research about the benefits of Sirtuins, there's little to no research about the specific Sirtfood diet. Besides, we already have some guidelines in place that have been thoroughly researched and tested for decades. If you're lost on what "healthy food" is, this is a better place to start».*

**My Opinion:** Well, the creators of this diet program are no spring chickens.

Aidan Goggins is a certified pharmacist and a certified nutritionist too. He has a Bachelor's degree in Pharmacy, and a Master's degree in Nutritional Science.

His partner, Glen Mattens, is also a certified nutritionist who is well known in the United Kingdom especially among celebrities.

Both of them are highly sought after by celebrities and athletes from all over the world.

Also, the research on the effects and benefits of Sirtuins especially for weight loss, are no secret, and has even been published in various medical journals in the past.

Sirtuin-activating compounds are also common knowledge in the food and medical industry and there have been many research programme funded by industry leaders to find out more about these compounds.

So, when people keep saying the Sirtfood diet is not backed by science, I get confused.

Are Sirtuins real and do they exist in the human body? Yes. Does SIRT 1 help to boost metabolic rate in the body? Yes. Are there foods that contain Sirtuin-activating compounds? Yes

So, what more 'scientific backing' do we need?

- **The Sirtfood Diet Can Damage Your Relationship with Food: On their website, they said:** *«This diet emphasizes an intake of 1,000 to 1,500 calories per day, which is much lower than most people need. When we severely limit our food intake, our instinctive reaction is to overeat. Your body is smart, and it considers this lack of sustenance as an attack. Therefore, we tend to overcompensate, which is why we all can relate to being "han-*

gry" and consequently overindulging when we're finally given a chance to eat. Practicing mindful and intuitive eating is a more sustainable route than restricting food."

My Opinion: Okay, this just confirms that they just read about the diet on some blog and quickly threw a criticism together.

A 7-day calorie restriction will not damage your relationship with food. Like I said, it's just a simple 'detox' to get your body introduced to Sirtuin-activating compounds and correct the negative effects that unhealthy eating habits have had on your body over the years.

## Getting started

There are a few things you have to put in place in order to ensure that the diet goes smoothly for you.

- Buy a Juicer: You will be having a lot of juice on this diet so make sure you get yourself a juicer. But if you can't afford one, here's a way to make your juices until you can get a juicer:

Step One: Add all the ingredients to your blender and process until smooth.

Step Two: Place a mesh cloth inside a bowl and pour the pulp from the blender into the mesh cloth. Squeeze the mesh cloth until you get all of the juice out into the bowl.

Step Three: Add ice and enjoy your juice.

- Get Organized: Plan all your meals for each week ahead. Go through each recipe and check your food storage to be sure you have all the ingredients and supplies you will need for each meal. This helps to ensure that you stay on track throughout the diet.
- Meal Prepping: It helps to look at your to-do list and see how busy your week might be. If you're going to have a busy week, you should consider meal prepping.

Cook your main meals during the weekend or a day ahead and store them in your refrigerator, so that you can simply reheat and enjoy.

It's best to have fresh juice but if you lead a busy life, it's okay to make the next day's juice a night before, refrigerate, take and go.

- Plan Your Meal Times: You would also need to schedule your meal times ahead, you know why? Because you must have your Sirt juice at least an hour before any main meal.

And remember, you must have finished eating all of your meals for the day by 7PM, so that means if your one main meal for the day is dinner, you must have had your Sirt juice by 6pm at most.

- Don't Obsess: I know that when you are on a diet, you would often feel the need to check the scales regularly to see how much weight you've lost but the creators of the Sirtfood diet have advised against this.

Weight loss goes beyond scale measurements- a lot of things begin to happen in your body as soon as you begin the diet and some of these results may not show up on a scale until the last few days of the diet (the 7-day phase).

So, if you keep running to the scales every time, you may get discouraged before your body has had time to adjust to the full effects of the diet.

- Drink Enough Water: Lastly, make sure you are drinking enough water daily. You should drink at least 2 liters of water every day as it helps your body flush out the toxins that will be dislodged as old fatty cells begin to burn up as fat.

# Breakfast Recipes

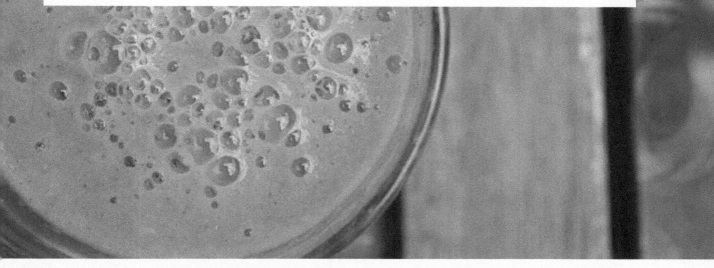

# Sirtfood Green Juice

## INGREDIENTS (FOR 1 SERVINGS)

- 75 g kale
- 30 g arugula
- 5 g flat-leaf parsley
- 2 large celery stalks with leaves
- 1/2 medium green apple
- 1 1-inch piece of fresh ginger
- juice of 1/2 lemon
- 1/2 level tsp. Matcha powder

## COOKING DIRECTIONS

1. Add celery, arugula, parsley, and kale to your juicer and extract the juice.
2. Add green apples and ginger, juice separately.
3. Squeeze in juice of 1/2 lemon.
4. Stir in Matcha powder.
5. Serve.

# Bunless Beef burgers

## INGREDIENTS (FOR 1 SERVINGS)

- 10 g arugula
- 125 g lean minced beef
- 30 g tomato (sliced)
- 15 g red onion (finely chopped)
- 10 g cheddar cheese (grated)
- 150 g sweet potatoes (cut into 1cm thick chips)
- 1 gherkin
- 1 garlic clove (unpeeled)
- 1 tsp. dried rosemary
- 1 tsp. Extra virgin olive oil
- 1 tsp. parsley (finely chopped)
- 15 g red onion (finely chopped)

## COOKING DIRECTIONS

1. Preheat your oven 220 C/ 428 F.
2. Drizzle potato chips with olive oil, garlic cloves, and rosemary.
3. Spread the chips on a baking sheet and roast in the oven for 30 minutes. Set aside
4. Combine parsley, onion and minced beef. Mix together and mold into a burger with your hands.
5. Place a frying pan over medium heat and add olive oil to heat up.
6. Place the burger on one side of a pan, and the onion rings on the other side of the pan. Let the burger cook for 6 minutes.
7. Fry onion rings as the burger cooks.
8. When the burger is cooked through, remove it from the oven and place on a baking tray. Top with onion rings and cheese.
9. Place in the oven and cook until cheese melts.
10. Serve with a mixture of gherkin, arugula and tomato and with fries on the side.

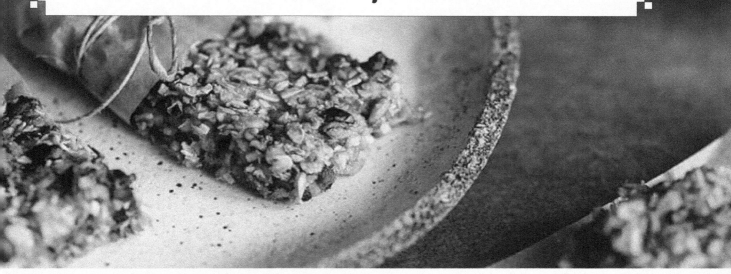

# Chocolate Chip Granola

## INGREDIENTS (FOR 8 SERVINGS)

- 60 g good-quality (70%) dark chocolate chips
- 200 g jumbo oats
- 20 g butter
- 50 g pecans (roughly chopped)
- 2 tbsp. of rice malt syrup
- 3 tbsp. light olive oil
- 1 tbsp. of dark brown sugar

## COOKING DIRECTIONS

1. Pre-heat your oven to 160C/320F.
2. Line a large baking tray with parchment paper.
3. Combine pecans and oats in a bowl and mix together.
4. Place a small non-stick pan over heat, and add olive oil, brown sugar, butter, and rice malt syrup. Let everything melt together and then stir. Make sure it doesn't boil.
5. Pour the mixture over your pecans and oats. Stir thoroughly.
6. Pour everything inside the baking tray and spread evenly.
7. Place in the oven to bake for 20 minutes.
8. Remove it from the oven and let it cool down
9. Break the granola into smaller clumps.
10. Store in an airtight jar.

# *Strawberry Buckwheat Tabbouleh*

## INGREDIENTS (FOR 1 SERVINGS)

- 30 g arugula
- 50 g buckwheat
- 100 g strawberries (hulled)
- 80 g avocado
- 30 g parsley
- 65 g tomato
- 25 g Medjool dates (pitted)
- 20 g red onion
- Juice of 1/2 lemon
- 1 tbsp. of ground turmeric
- 1 tbsp. Extra virgin olive oil
- 1 tbsp. of capers

## COOKING DIRECTIONS

1. Add turmeric to the buckwheat and cook according to the instructions on the package.
2. Drain and set aside.
3. Chop and mix parsley, avocado, capers, tomatoes, red onions, and dates.
4. Slice strawberries and add it to the mixture.
5. Add cooked buckwheat and stir.
6. Drizzle with lemon juice and olive oil.
7. Serve over bed of arugula.

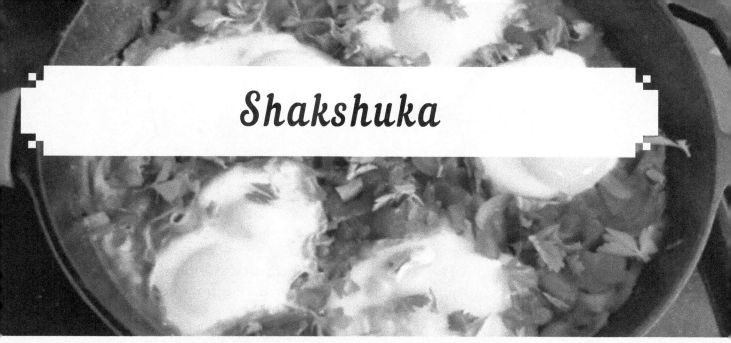

# Shakshuka

## INGREDIENTS (FOR 1 SERVINGS)

- 30 g kale (stems removed and roughly chopped)
- 40 g red onion (finely chopped)
- 400 g canned chopped tomatoes
- 30 g celery (finely chopped)
- 2 medium eggs
- 1 garlic clove (finely chopped)

- 1 tsp. of paprika
- 1 tsp. of ground cumin
- 1 Bird's eye chili (finely chopped)
- 1 tsp. ground turmeric
- 1 tbsp. of chopped parsley
- 1 tsp. of Extra virgin olive oil

## COOKING DIRECTIONS

1. Place a deep-sided frying pan over medium heat and add olive oil to heat up.
2. Fry your garlic, onion, chili, celery, and all your spices in the pan for 2 minutes.
3. Add tomatoes and stir. Let it simmer for 20 minutes, making sure to stir every 5 minutes.
4. Add kale and some water to thin out the sauce if necessary. Let it simmer for another 5 minutes.
5. Add parsley and stir.
6. Use your spoon to make two holes in between the sauce, and crack one egg into each hole.
7. Reduce the heat further, and then cover the pan with foil paper.
8. Leave to cook for 10 minutes.
9. The Shakshuka is ready the egg yolks and egg white are firm and well cooked.
10. Serve.

# Date and Walnut Loaf

## INGREDIENTS (FOR 1 SERVINGS)

- 30 g arugula
- 50 g buckwheat
- 100 g strawberries (hulled)
- 80 g avocado
- 30 g parsley
- 65 g tomato
- 25 g Medjool dates (pitted)
- 20 g red onion
- Juice of 1/2 lemon
- 1 tbsp. of ground turmeric
- 1 tbsp. Extra virgin olive oil
- 1 tbsp. of capers

## COOKING DIRECTIONS

1. Add turmeric to the buckwheat and cook according to the instructions on the package.
2. Drain and set aside.
3. Chop and mix parsley, avocado, capers, tomatoes, red onions, and dates.
4. Slice strawberries and add it to the mixture.
5. Add cooked buckwheat and stir.
6. Drizzle with lemon juice and olive oil.
7. Serve over bed of arugula.

# Moroccan Spiced Eggs

## INGREDIENTS (FOR 1 SERVINGS)

- 400 g canned chopped tomatoes
- 10 g flat-leaf parsley chopped
- 400 g canned chickpeas
- 1 tsp. of olive oil
- 4 medium eggs (room temperature)
- 1 shallot (peeled and finely chopped)
- 1/2 tsp. of salt
- 1 red bell pepper (deseeded and finely chopped)
- 1/4 tsp. of ground cumin
- 1 garlic clove (peeled and finely chopped)
- 1/4 tsp. of ground cinnamon
- 1 zucchini (peeled and finely chopped)
- 1/2 tsp. of mild chili powder
- 1 tbsp. of tomato paste

## COOKING DIRECTIONS

1. Place a saucepan over high heat and add oil to heat up.
2. Add red bell pepper and shallots to the oil and fry for 6 minutes.
3. Add zucchini and stir. Let it cook for 1 minute.
4. Add all your spices, salt, and tomato puree. Stir and let it cook for 2 minutes.
5. Add chickpeas along with the canning water and stir.
6. Add chopped tomatoes and stir.
7. Increase the heat and allow the sauce simmer for 30 minutes.
8. Pre-heat your oven to 180C/350 F.
9. Reduce the heat of the tomato sauce and bring the sauce to a gentle simmer.
10. Pour the sauce in your baking dish.
11. Crack eggs into the sides of the baking dish (into the sauce but on the sides)
12. Cover the baking dish with foil paper and place it in your oven to cook for 15 minutes.
13. Serve.

# Iced Cranberry Green Tea

## INGREDIENTS (FOR 1 SERVINGS)

- Handful of crushed ice
- 150 ml cranberry juice
- A squeeze of lemon
- A sprig of mint
- 100 ml of green tea (room temperature)

## COOKING DIRECTIONS

1. Add all ingredients to a glass cup and garnish with mint leaf.
2. Serve.

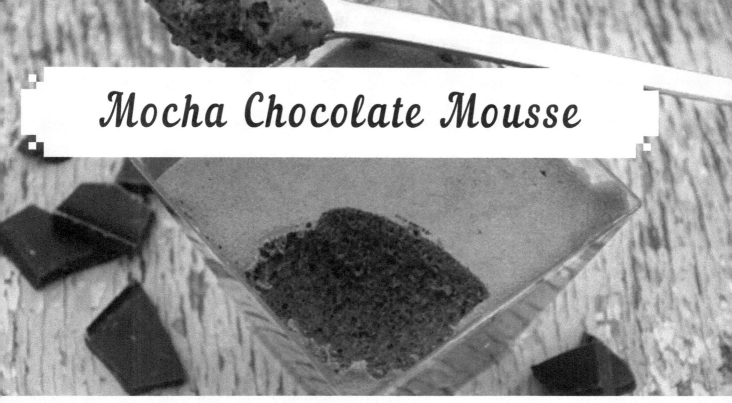

# Mocha Chocolate Mousse

## INGREDIENTS (FOR 4 SERVINGS)

- 250 g dark chocolate (85% cocoa solids)
- 4 tbsp. of almond milk
- 6 free-range eggs (separate yolk from egg whites)
- Chocolate coffee beans
- 4 tbsp. of strong black coffee

## COOKING DIRECTIONS

1. Place a pot over medium heat, add water and bring to a boil. Reduce heat to low.
2. Place a stainless-steel bowl over the boiling water (don't let the bottom of the bowl touch the water) and add chocolate to melt.
3. Remove melted chocolate from heat and let it cool down to room temperature.
4. Add the yolk of one egg at a time and whisk as you add.
5. Fold almond milk and coffee in gently.
6. Whisk the egg whites with a hand-held electric mixer until a stiff peak forms.
7. Incorporate the chocolate mixture into the egg whites one tablespoon at a time while using the electric mixer to continue to mix it.
8. Transfer to serving glasses covered with cling film. Leave in the refrigerator to chill overnight.
9. Serve with coffee beans on top.

# Ginger and Turmeric Tea

## INGREDIENTS (FOR 1 SERVINGS)

- A cup of hot water
- 1-inch piece of fresh ginger (peeled)
- 1 tsp. of honey
- 1/4 tsp. of turmeric

## COOKING DIRECTIONS

1. Use a knife to make holes in the ginger and add it to a tea cup.
2. Add turmeric and add hot water.
3. Let it infuse for 8 minutes.
4. Serve.

# Buckwheat Superfood Muesli

## INGREDIENTS (FOR 1 SERVINGS)

- 100 g plain Greek yogurt or coconut yogurt
- 20 g buckwheat flakes
- 100 g strawberries (chopped)
- 10 g buckwheat puffs
- 10 g cocoa nibs
- 15 g coconut flakes
- 15 g walnuts (chopped)
- 40 g Medjool dates (pitted and chopped)

## COOKING DIRECTIONS

1. Combine all ingredients (except yogurt and strawberries) in a serving bowl. Mix.
2. Serve topped with strawberries and yogurt.

# Ginger and Turmeric Tea

## INGREDIENTS (FOR 1 SERVINGS)

- A cup of hot water
- 1-inch piece of fresh ginger (peeled)
- 1 tsp. of honey
- 1/4 tsp. of turmeric

## COOKING DIRECTIONS

1. Use a knife to make holes in the ginger and add it to a tea cup.
2. Add turmeric and add hot water.
3. Let it infuse for 8 minutes.
4. Serve.

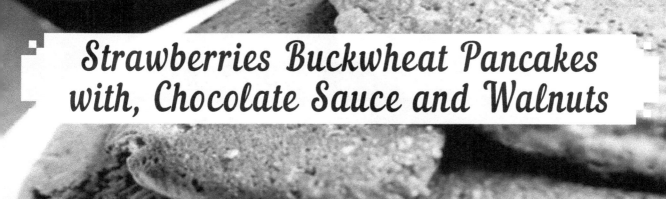

# Strawberries Buckwheat Pancakes with, Chocolate Sauce and Walnuts

## INGREDIENTS (FOR 1 SERVINGS)

For Chocolate Sauce:
- 1 tbsp. of double cream
- 100 g of dark chocolate (85% cocoa solids)
- 1 tbsp. of Extra virgin olive oil
- 85 ml of milk

For Pancakes:
- 150 g of buckwheat flour
- 1 tbsp. of Extra virgin olive oil
- 350 ml milk
- 1 large egg

For Serving:
- 100 g walnuts (chopped)
- 400 g strawberries (hulled and chopped)

## COOKING DIRECTIONS

1. Start by making your pancake batter. Add all the ingredients for the pancakes (except the olive oil) to your blender and process until it forms a smooth batter.
2. Place a heavy-bottomed frying pan over medium heat.
3. When the pan starts to smoke, add olive oil to heat up, and then scoop some of the batter into the pan. Cook until it starts to bubble at the top, flip and then cook the other side for a minute.
4. Repeat the process until you've exhausted all your pancake batter.
5. Now, make your chocolate sauce. Place a heatproof bowl over a pan of simmering hot water. Add chocolate to the bowl to melt.
6. Whisk in the olive oil, milk, and double cream until it is well incorporated.
7. Serve sauce over pancakes.
8. Sprinkle walnuts over sauce.

# Black Forest Smoothie

## INGREDIENTS (FOR 1 SERVINGS)

- 200 ml of soy milk
- 100 g of frozen cherries
- 2 tsp. of chia seeds
- 25 g of kale
- 1 tbsp. of cocoa powder
- 1 Medjool date

## COOKING DIRECTIONS

1. Combine all ingredients in your blender and process until smooth.
2. Serve.

# Blueberry Banana Pancakes with Chunky Apple Compote and Golden Turmeric Latte

## INGREDIENTS (FOR 1 SERVINGS)

For Chunky Apple Compote:
- 1 tbsp. of lemon juice
- 2 apples (cored and roughly chopped)
- Pinch of salt
- 5 dates (pitted)
- 1/4 tsp. of cinnamon powder

For Blueberry Banana Pancakes:
- 25 g blueberries
- 150g rolled oats
- 1/4 tsp. of salt
- 6 eggs
- 2 tsp. of baking powder
- 6 bananas

For Golden Turmeric Latte:
- 1 tsp. of cinnamon powder
- 3 cups coconut milk
- Pinch of cayenne pepper
- 1 tsp. of turmeric powder
- Pinch of black pepper
- 1 tsp. raw honey
- Fresh, peeled ginger root (tiny piece, fresh)

## COOKING DIRECTIONS

1. Pulse rolled oats in your blender for a minute until it turns into flour. Pour the flour into a bowl and set aside.
2. Now, add bananas along with baking powder, eggs and salt to the blender and pulse for 2 minutes. Pour the banana mixture into the flour and mix well to form a smooth batter.
3. Fold blueberries in.
4. Set batter aside.
5. Place a frying pan over heat and add a dollop of butter to melt and heat up.
6. Scoop pancake batter into the pan and cook until the pancakes start to sizzle. Flip and cook for another 2 minutes.
7. Set cook pancakes aside to make apple compote.
8. Add apples to your food processor.
9. Add a pinch of salt, lemon juice, pitted dates, Cinnamon powder, and 2 tablespoons of water. Pulse until it forms chunky apple compote. Set aside.
10. Add all ingredients for the turmeric latte to the blender and process until smooth.
11. Place a small saucepan over medium heat and then pour the mixture into it and cook it for 4 minutes.
12. Combine all the elements and serve.

# Mushroom and Buckwheat Pancakes

## INGREDIENTS (FOR 2 SERVINGS)

- 1 red onion (chopped)
- 125 g buckwheat flour
- 1 tsp. of olive oil
- 1 egg
- 150 ml of water
- 150 ml of semi-skimmed milk

## COOKING DIRECTIONS

1. Sift buckwheat flour into a bowl.
2. Crack eggs into the bowl and mix with buckwheat flour.
3. Add water and milk and mix.
4. Let it sit for 5 minutes.
5. Place a pan over heat and add olive oil to heat up.
6. Add mushrooms and onions to the pan. Sauté for 5 minutes.
7. Add spinach and cook until they wilt.
8. Remove from heat and set aside.
9. Place a frying pan over medium heat and add a teaspoon of olive oil to heat up.
10. Scoop 1/4 cup of batter into the frying pan. Cook for 2 minutes.
11. Flip and cook the other side for 1 minute.
12. Remove from heat and repeat until you've exhausted the pancake batter.
13. Serve pancake over a bed of arugula leaves and top with mushrooms and spinach mix.

# Blueberry Smoothie

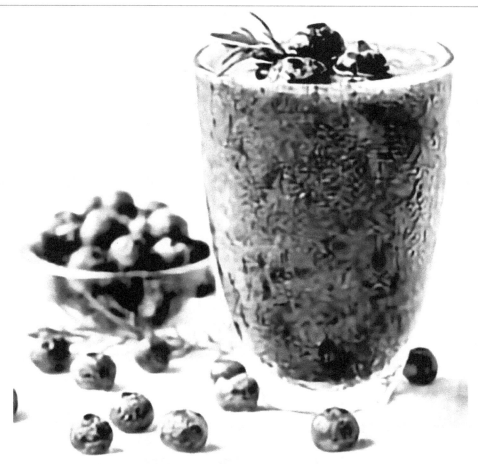

## INGREDIENTS (FOR 2 SERVINGS)

- 100 g blackberries
- 200 ml of milk
- 100 g blueberries
- 2 tbsp. of natural yogurt
- 1 ripe banana

## COOKING DIRECTIONS

1. Combine all ingredients in your blender or food processor.
2. Process until smooth.

# Herb and Olives Frittata

## INGREDIENTS (FOR 2 SERVINGS)

- 1 tbsp. of olive oil
- 50 g cheddar cheese
- 1 tsp. of fresh basil (chopped)
- 1 tbsp. of fresh parsley(chopped)

- 4 large eggs
- 8 cherry tomatoes (halved)
- 75 g black olives (pitted)

## COOKING DIRECTIONS

1. Crack the eggs into a mixing bowl.
2. Add tomatoes, parsley, olives and basil, and whisk together.
3. Add cheese and whisk some more.
4. Place a frying pan over medium heat and add olive oil to heat up.
5. Pour the egg mixture inside and stir until scrambled and then serve.

# Turmeric Pancakes with Lemon Yogurt Sauce

## INGREDIENTS (FOR 4 SERVINGS)

For Pancakes:
- 3 large eggs (lightly beaten)
- 2 tsp. of ground turmeric
- 4 tsp. of coconut oil
- 11/2 tsp. of ground cumin
- 1 cup of almond flour
- 1 tsp. of salt
- 2 tbsp. of plain unsweetened almond milk
- 1 tsp. of ground coriander
- 1 head of broccoli (cut into florets)
- 1/2 tsp. of garlic powder
- 1/2 tsp. of freshly ground black pepper

For Yogurt Sauce:
- 1 garlic clove (minced)
- 2 tsp. of lemon zest (from 1 lemon)
- 1 cup of plain Greek yogurt
- 10 fresh mint leaves (minced)
- 2 tbsp. of lemon juice
- 1/4 tsp. of ground turmeric

## COOKING DIRECTIONS

1. Add lemon juice, garlic, turmeric, yogurt, zest, and mint to a mixing bowl. Mix well.

2. Let it sit in the refrigerator until your pancakes are ready.

3. Combine garlic, pepper, coriander, salt, cumin and turmeric in another bowl and mix well.

4. Add broccoli florets to a food processor and process until a bit smooth. Pour into a bowl.

5. Add almond flour, almond milk, eggs, and the turmeric mixture into the broccoli mixture and stir until well incorporated.

6. Place a non-stick frying pan over medium heat and add coconut oil to heat up.

7. Scoop 1/4 cup of the batter into the pan and cook until bubbles form at the top of your pancakes.

8. Flip and cook the other side for a minute.

9. Repeat until you've exhausted all of your pancake batter.

10. Serve pancakes with yogurt sauce.

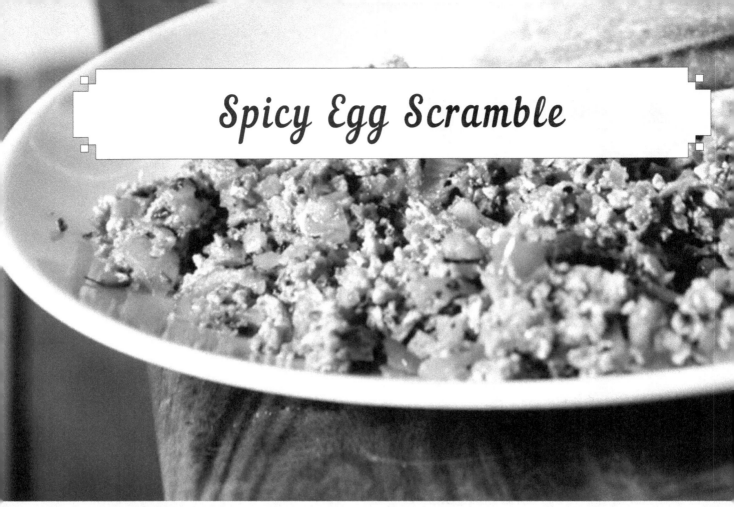

# Spicy Egg Scramble

## INGREDIENTS (FOR 1 SERVINGS)

- 2 eggs
- 25 g kale (finely chopped)
- Sea salt and freshly ground black pepper to taste
- 1 tsp. of turmeric
- 1 scallion
- 1 tbsp. of olive oil

## COOKING DIRECTIONS

1. 2 eggs
2. 25 g kale (finely chopped)
3. Sea salt and freshly ground black pepper to taste
4. 1 tsp. of turmeric
5. 1 scallion
6. 1 tbsp. of olive oil

# Grape and Melon Juice

## INGREDIENTS (FOR 1 SERVINGS)

- 100 g cantaloupe melon (peeled, deseeded and cut into chunks)
- 100 g red seedless grapes
- 30 g young spinach leaves (stalks removed)
- 1/2 cucumber (peeled, halved, seeds removed and roughly chopped)

## COOKING DIRECTIONS

1. Combine all ingredients into your juicer or blender, and blend until smooth.
2. Serve.

# Veggie Egg Scramble

## INGREDIENTS (FOR 1 SERVINGS)

- 1 tbsp. of olive oil
- 2 eggs
- 1 tbsp. of olive oil
- 25 g of arugula

- 1 tsp. of fresh parsley
- 1 tsp. of fresh basil
- 1 tsp. of chives
- Sea salt and black pepper to taste

## COOKING DIRECTIONS

1. Crack the eggs into a small bowl and whisk.
2. Crack the eggs into a mixing bowl.
3. Add all other ingredients and whisk together.
4. Place a frying pan over medium heat and add olive oil to heat up.
5. Pour the egg mixture inside and stir until scrambled.
6. Add black pepper and sea salt to taste.
7. Serve.

# Kale and Blackcurrant Smoothie

## INGREDIENTS (FOR 2 SERVINGS)

- 40 g blackcurrants (washed and stalks removed)
- 2 tsp. of honey
- 6 ice cubes
- 1 ripe banana
- 10 baby kale leaves (stalks removed)
- 1 cup of freshly made green tea

## COOKING DIRECTIONS

1. Add honey to the freshly made green tea and stir.
2. Add all other ingredients along with your green tea mixture into your blender and pulse until smooth.
3. Serve.

# Cheesy Baked Eggs

## INGREDIENTS (FOR 1 SERVINGS)

- 1 tbsp. of parsley
- 4 large eggs
- 1 tbsp. of olive oil
- 75 g grated cheese
- 1/2 tsp. ground turmeric
- 25 g fresh arugula

## COOKING DIRECTIONS

1. Pre-heat your oven to 220C/400F.
2. Coat 4 ramekin dishes with olive oil.
3. Add a bed of arugula leaves in each ramekin dish and crack an egg into each of them.
4. Sprinkle cheese, turmeric, and parsley on top of each ramekin dish.
5. Bake in the oven for 15 minutes; serve.

# Buckwheat Pasta Salad

## INGREDIENTS (FOR 1 SERVINGS)

- 20 g pine nuts
- 50 g buckwheat pasta (cooked according to the packet instructions)
- 1 tbsp. of Extra virgin olive oil
- Large handful of arugula
- 1 tbsp. of Extra virgin olive oil
- Small handful of basil leaves
- 10 olives
- 1/2 avocado (diced)
- 8 cherry tomatoes (halved)

## COOKING DIRECTIONS

1. Mix all ingredients except pine nuts together in a salad bowl.
2. Garnish with pine nuts.

# Crunchy Fruit and Nut Yoghurt

## INGREDIENTS (FOR 1 SERVINGS)

- 50 g strawberries (chopped)
- A pinch of cocoa powder
- 100 g plain Greek yogurt
- 3 walnuts (halved)

## COOKING DIRECTIONS

1. Pour the yogurt into a cereal bowl.
2. Add walnuts and strawberries and mix.
3. Garnish with a pinch of cocoa powder.
4. Serve.

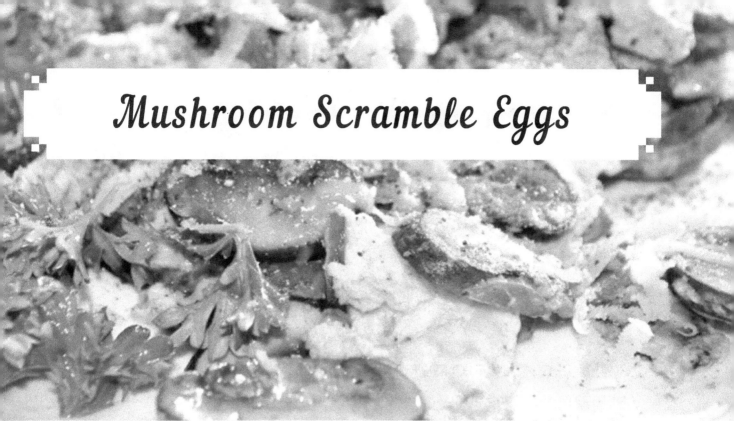

# Mushroom Scramble Eggs

## INGREDIENTS (FOR 1 SERVINGS)

- 5 g parsley (finely chopped)
- 20 g kale (roughly chopped)
- Handful of button mushrooms, thinly sliced
- 2 eggs
- 1/2 Bird's eye chili, thinly sliced
- 1 tsp. of ground turmeric
- 1 tsp. of Extra virgin olive oil
- 1 tsp. of mild curry powder

## COOKING DIRECTIONS

1. Combine curry powder and turmeric in a bowl and add a little bit of water to form a light paste.
2. Place a pot of water over heat and bring to a boil. Steam kale in the boiling water for 3 minutes. Drain and set aside.
3. Place a frying pan over medium heat and add oil to heat up. Then add mushrooms and chili, fry for 3 minutes.
4. Add curry paste and stir.
5. Add steamed kale and stir.
6. Crack eggs into a bowl and whisk together.
7. Pour eggs into the frying pan and scramble.
8. Serve.

# Walnut and Strawberry Porridge

## INGREDIENTS (FOR 1 SERVINGS)

- 100 ml water
- 100 g strawberries
- 1 cup of unsweetened soya milk
- 50 g rolled oats
- 1 tsp. of chia seeds
- 2 walnuts (chopped in halves)

## COOKING DIRECTIONS

1. Combine soy milk, strawberries, oats, and water in your blender and blend until smooth.
2. Add chia seeds and mix.
3. Let it sit in the refrigerator overnight.
4. Sprinkle chopped walnuts all over it.
5. Serve

# Smoked Salmon Omelet

## INGREDIENTS (FOR 1 SERVINGS)

- 10 g arugula (chopped)
- 100 g smoked salmon (sliced)
- 1 tsp. of Extra virgin olive oil
- 2 medium eggs
- 1 tsp. of parsley (chopped)
- 1/2 tsp. of capers

## COOKING DIRECTIONS

1. Break your eggs into a bowl and whisk well.
2. Add parsley, carpers, arugula, and salmon to the eggs and continue to whisk until everything is well incorporated.
3. Place a nonstick frying pan over medium heat and add oil to heat up.
4. Pour the egg mixture into the pan and let it cook through and serve.

# Nutty Strawberry Breakfast Granola

## INGREDIENTS (FOR 4 SERVINGS)

- 100 g almonds (chopped)
- 250 g buckwheat flakes
- 200 g oats
- 1/2 cup olive oil
- 250 g buckwheat flour

- 2 tbsp. honey
- 100 g dried strawberry
- 100 g walnuts (chopped)
- 1 1/2 tsp. of ground cinnamon
- 1 1/2 tsp. of ground ginger

## COOKING DIRECTIONS

1. Preheat your oven to 150C / 300F.
2. Pour the nuts into a bowl and add oats, ginger, buckwheat flakes, cinnamon, and nuts. Mix everything together.
3. Pour olive oil into a saucepan placed over heat.
4. Add honey to the pan and stir.
5. When the honey and olive oil is melted and well mixed together, pour it inside the cinnamon and oats mixture. Mix well.
6. Pour everything on a large baking tray and spread it well.
7. Bake in the oven for 50 minutes.
8. Bring it out and allow it cool down.
9. Mix your dried berries in.
10. Store in an airtight container or serve immediately.

# Green Tea Smoothie

## INGREDIENTS (FOR 2 SERVINGS)

- 2 tsp. of honey
- 1/2 tsp. of vanilla bean paste
- 2 ripe bananas
- 6 ice cubes
- 2 tsp. of Matcha green tea powder
- 250 ml milk

## COOKING DIRECTIONS

1. Combine all ingredients in a blender and process until smooth.
2. Serve.

# *Strawberry and Buckwheat Pancakes*

## INGREDIENTS (FOR 4 SERVINGS)

- 100 g of strawberries
- 2 tsp. of olive oil
- 100 g buckwheat
- 250 ml milk
- 1 egg
- Freshly squeezed orange juice

## COOKING DIRECTIONS

1. Crack eggs into a bowl.
2. Add the milk and 1 tsp. of olive oil. Whisk until well combined.
3. Add the flour and mix.
4. Let it sit for 20 minutes.
5. Add strawberries to the batter and mix.
6. Place a pan over medium heat and add another tsp. of oil.
7. When the oil is hot enough scoop 1/4 cup of the batter into the pan.
8. Let it cook for 2 minutes.
9. Flip and cook the second side for another minute.
10. Repeat until your batter is exhausted.
11. Serve with freshly squeezed orange juice.

# Summer Berry Smoothie

## INGREDIENTS (FOR 1 SERVINGS)

- Juice of 1 lime
- 50 g strawberries
- 1 orange (peeled)
- 50 g blueberries
- 1 carrot (peeled)
- 25 g red grapes
- 25 g blackcurrants

## COOKING DIRECTIONS

1. Combine all ingredients in your blender and add a little water to cover the ingredients.
2. Add ice cubes or crushed ice to taste.
3. Blend until smooth.
4. Serve.

# Sirtfood Poached Eggs

## INGREDIENTS (FOR 1 SERVINGS)

- 25 g fresh arugula leaves
- 2 eggs
- Sea salt and freshly ground black pepper to taste
- 1 tsp. of olive oil

## COOKING DIRECTIONS

1. Pour the arugula leaves into a plate.
2. Sprinkle the olive oil all over the leaves.
3. Place a shallow pan over heat and water to boil.
4. Crack the eggs inside the water and let it cook until the egg whites are firm.
5. Transfer the eggs into serving dishes and add the arugula leaves on top of it.
6. Sprinkle with salt and pepper and serve.

# Sirtfood Cocktail

## INGREDIENTS (FOR 1 SERVINGS)

- A squeeze of lemon juice
- 75 g kale
- 1 tsp. Matcha powder
- 50 g strawberries
- 1 tbsp. of parsley
- 1 apple (cored)
- 2 sticks of celery

## COOKING DIRECTIONS

1. Combine all ingredients in your blender and add a little water to cover the ingredients.
2. Add ice cubes or crushed ice to taste.
3. Blend until smooth.
4. Serve.

# Arugula and Mango Blitz

## INGREDIENTS (FOR 1 SERVINGS)

- Juice of 1 lime
- 25 g of arugula
- 1/2 tsp. of Matcha powder
- 150 g of mango (peeled, deseeded, chopped)
- 1 avocado (peeled and deseeded)

## COOKING DIRECTIONS

1. Combine all ingredients in your blender and add a little water to cover the ingredients.
2. Add ice cubes or crushed ice to taste
3. Blend until smooth.
4. Serve.

# Grape, Celery, and Mango Smoothie

## INGREDIENTS (FOR 1 SERVINGS)

- 50 g kale
- 50 g mango (peeled, deseeded, chopped)
- 1-inch piece of fresh ginger (peeled and chopped)
- 1 stalk of celery
- 1 apple (cored)

## COOKING DIRECTIONS

1. Combine all ingredients in your blender and add a little water.
2. Add ice cubes or crushed ice to taste.
3. Blend until smooth.
4. Serve.

# Kale and Cranberry Smoothie

## INGREDIENTS (FOR 1 SERVINGS)

- 1 tsp. of chia seeds
- 75 g of strawberries
- 1/2 tsp. of Matcha powder
- 1/2 cup of unsweetened cranberry juice
- 50 g kale
- One fresh mint leaf

## COOKING DIRECTIONS

1. Combine all ingredients in your blender and add a little water to cover the ingredients.
2. Add ice cubes or crushed ice to taste.
3. Blend until smooth.
4. Serve.

# Kale, Carrot, and Orange Smoothie

## INGREDIENTS (FOR 1 SERVINGS)

- 50 g kale
- 1 carrot (peeled)
- 1/2 tsp. Matcha powder
- 1 orange (peeled)
- 1 apple (cored)
- 1 stick of celery

## COOKING DIRECTIONS

1. Combine all ingredients in your blender and add a little water to cover the ingredients.
2. Add ice cubes or crushed ice to taste.
3. Blend until smooth.
4. Serve.

# Berry Blend

## INGREDIENTS (FOR 1 SERVINGS)

- 50 g strawberries
- 50 g blueberries
- 50 g kale
- 1 cup of unsweetened soya milk
- 1 tbsp. of cocoa powder
- 1 banana

## COOKING DIRECTIONS

1. Combine all ingredients in your blender.
2. Add ice cubes or crushed ice to taste
3. Blend until smooth.
4. Serve.

# Cherry and Creamy Berry Smoothie

## INGREDIENTS (FOR 1 SERVINGS)

- 1 tbsp. of plain full fat yogurt
- 100 g strawberries
- 175 ml unsweetened soya milk
- 75 g pitted dates

## COOKING DIRECTIONS

1. Combine all ingredients in your blender and pulse until smooth and creamy.
2. Serve.

# Coconut, Strawberry and Chocolate Smoothie

## INGREDIENTS (FOR 1 SERVINGS)

- 1 tsp. of Matcha powder
- 100 ml coconut milk
- 1 tbsp. of cocoa powder
- 1 banana
- 100 g strawberries

## COOKING DIRECTIONS

1. Combine all ingredients in your blender.
2. Add ice cubes or crushed ice to taste
3. Blend until creamy and smooth.
4. Add a little water while blending to thin out the smoothie if you wish.
5. Serve.

# Celery Grape and Parsley Blitz

## INGREDIENTS (FOR 1 SERVINGS)

- 1 tbsp. of fresh parsley
- 75 g of red grapes
- 1/2 tsp. of Matcha
- 1 avocado (deseeded and peeled)
- 3 sticks of celery

## COOKING DIRECTIONS

1. Combine all ingredients in your blender and add a little water to cover the ingredients.
2. Add ice cubes or crushed ice to taste.
3. Blend until smooth.
4. Serve.

# Ginger and Banana Blitz

## INGREDIENTS (FOR 1 SERVINGS)

- 1/4 tsp. of turmeric powder
- 1-inch chunk of fresh ginger (peeled)
- 1/2 stick of celery
- 1 apple (cored)
- 1 banana
- 1 carrot

## COOKING DIRECTIONS

1. Combine all ingredients in your blender and add a little water to cover the ingredients.
2. Add ice cubes or crushed ice to taste.
3. Blend until smooth.
4. Serve.

# Citrus and Strawberry Juice

## INGREDIENTS (FOR 1 SERVINGS)

- 1 avocado (deseeded and peeled)
- 1/2 tsp. Matcha powder
- 75 g of strawberries
- Juice of 1 lime
- 1 orange (peeled)
- 1 apple (peeled)

## COOKING DIRECTIONS

1. Combine all ingredients in your blender and add a little water to cover the ingredients.
2. Add ice cubes or crushed ice to taste.
3. Blend until smooth.
4. Serve.

# Pineapple, Avocado, Celery Smoothie

## INGREDIENTS (FOR 1 SERVINGS)

- Juice of 1 lemon
- 50 g fresh pineapple (peeled and chopped)
- 1/2 tsp. of Matcha powder
- 3 stalks of celery
- 1 tsp. of fresh parsley
- 1 avocado (peeled and deseeded)

## COOKING DIRECTIONS

1. Combine all ingredients in your blender and add a little water to cover the ingredients.
2. Add ice cubes or crushed ice to taste.
3. Blend until smooth.
4. Serve.

# Celery and Grapefruit Blitz

## INGREDIENTS (FOR 1 SERVINGS)

- 50 g of kale
- 1 grapefruit (peeled)
- 1/2 tsp. Matcha powder
- 2 stalks of celery

## COOKING DIRECTIONS

1. Combine all ingredients in your blender and add a little water to cover the ingredients.
2. Add ice cubes or crushed ice to taste.
3. Blend until smooth.
4. Serve.

# Tasty Arugula Smoothie

## INGREDIENTS (FOR 1 SERVINGS)

- 75 g of kale
- Juice of 1 lime
- 25 g of arugula
- 1 tbsp. of fresh parsley
- 1 carrot (peeled and chopped)
- 1 apple

## COOKING DIRECTIONS

1. Combine all ingredients in your blender and add a little water to cover the ingredients.
2. Add ice cubes or crushed ice to taste.
3. Blend until smooth.
4. Serve.

# Celery and Orange Blitz

## INGREDIENTS (FOR 1 SERVINGS)

- 1/2 tsp. Matcha powder
- Juice of 1 lime
- 3 stalks of celery
- 1 carrot (peeled)
- 1 orange (peeled)

## COOKING DIRECTIONS

1. Combine all ingredients in your blender and add a little water to cover the ingredients.
2. Add ice cubes or crushed ice to taste.
3. Blend until smooth.
4. Serve.

# Cucumber and Pineapple Blitz

## INGREDIENTS (FOR 1 SERVINGS)

- 50 g cucumber
- A squeeze of lemon juice
- 1 stalk of celery
- 1/2 tsp. of Matcha powder
- 2 sprigs of parsley
- 2 slices of pineapple

## COOKING DIRECTIONS

1. Combine all ingredients in your blender and add a little water to cover the ingredients.
2. Add ice cubes or crushed ice to taste.
3. Blend until smooth.
4. Serve

# Pineapple Chocolate Smoothie

## INGREDIENTS (FOR 1 SERVINGS)

- 75 g of fresh pineapple (chopped)
- 25 g arugula
- 50 g kale
- 1 mango (peeled and deseeded)
- 1/2 cup of coconut milk
- 1 tbsp. of cocoa powder

## COOKING DIRECTIONS

1. Combine all ingredients in your blender.
2. Add ice cubes or crushed ice to taste
3. Blend until creamy and smooth.
4. Add a little water while blending to thin out the smoothie if you wish.
5. Serve.

# Spiced Apples and Walnut Smoothie

## INGREDIENTS (FOR 1 SERVINGS)

- A pinch of ground nutmeg
- 6 walnut halves
- 1/2 tsp. Matcha powder
- 1/2 tsp. of cinnamon
- 1 banana
- 1 apple (cored)

## COOKING DIRECTIONS

1. Combine all ingredients in your blender and add a little water to cover the ingredients.
2. Add ice cubes or crushed ice to taste.
3. Blend until smooth.
4. Serve.

# Dates and Walnut Porridge

## INGREDIENTS (FOR 1 SERVINGS)

- 50 g strawberries (hulled)
- 200 ml milk
- 1 tsp. of walnut butter
- 1 Medjool date (chopped)
- 35 g buckwheat flakes

## COOKING DIRECTIONS

1. Place a saucepan over heat and add buckwheat flakes, dates, and milk. Cook for 2 minutes.
2. Add strawberries and stir.
3. Remove from heat.
4. Serve with walnut butter.

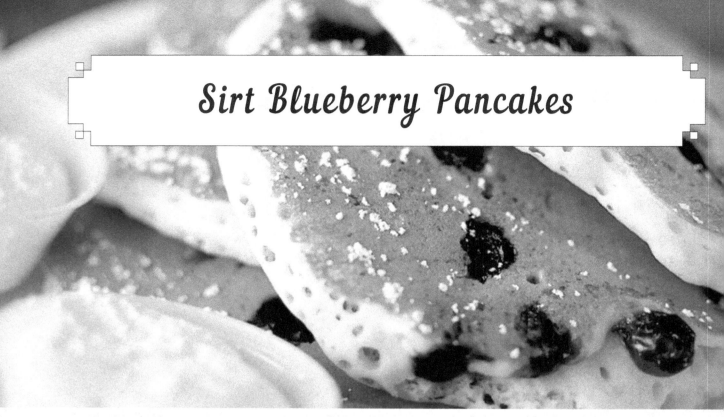

# Sirt Blueberry Pancakes

## INGREDIENTS (FOR 1 SERVINGS)

- 225 g blueberries
- 150 g rolled oats
- 1/4 tsp. salt
- 6 eggs
- 2 tsp. of baking powder
- 6 bananas

## COOKING DIRECTIONS

1. Pulse rolled oats in your blender for a minute until it turns into flour. Pour the flour into a bowl and set aside.
2. Add baking powder, eggs, and salt to the blender. Pulse for 2 minutes. Pour in a bowl and set aside.
3. Add bananas to the blender and blend into a paste.
4. Pour the banana mixture into the flour and mix well to form a smooth batter.
5. Fold blueberries in.
6. Set batter aside.
7. Place a frying pan over heat and some oil to coat the pan.
8. Scoop pancake batter into the pan and cook until the pancakes start to sizzle. Flip and cook for another 2 minutes.
9. Repeat until you've exhausted your batter.

# Lunch Recipes

# *Pomegranate Guacamole*

## INGREDIENTS (FOR 4 SERVINGS)

- Juice of 1 lime
- Flesh of 2 ripe avocados
- 1/2 red onion (finely chopped)
- 1 Bird's eye chili
- 1 pomegranate seed

## COOKING DIRECTIONS

1. Combine all ingredients in your blender or food process into a soft chunky mixture.
2. Serve.

# Braised Puy Lentils

## INGREDIENTS (FOR 1 SERVINGS)

- 20 g arugula
- 40 g red onion (thinly sliced)
- 50 g kale (roughly chopped)
- 75 g Puy lentils
- 40 g celery (thinly sliced)
- 8 cherry tomatoes (halved)
- 40 g carrots (peeled and thinly sliced)
- 1 tbsp. of parsley (chopped)
- 2 tsp. of Extra virgin olive oil
- 220 ml vegetable stock
- 1 tsp. of dried thyme
- 1 garlic clove (finely chopped)
- 1 tsp. of paprika

## COOKING DIRECTIONS

1. Preheat your oven to 120C/240 F.
2. Roast tomato in the oven for about 40 minutes.
3. Place a saucepan over low heat and add a tsp. of olive oil.
4. When the olive oil is hot enough, add garlic, carrots, celery, and red onion. Sauté until softened.
5. Add thyme and paprika. Cook for another minute.
6. Pour lentils in a fine-mesh sieve to drain before adding it to the pan.
7. Stir, and then bring to a boil.
8. Reduce the heat then allow it to simmer for 25 minutes while stirring every 5 minutes. You can add more water if necessary.
9. Add kale and cook for another 7 minutes.
10. Check to see if the lentils are well-cooked and if so, add roasted tomatoes and parsley. Stir.
11. Drizzle arugula with a tsp. of olive oil and serve with braised lentils.

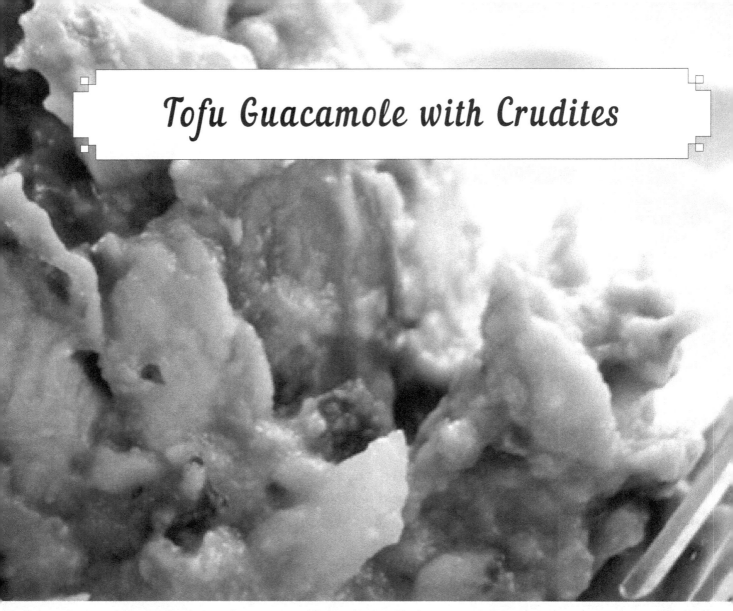

# Tofu Guacamole with Crudites

## INGREDIENTS (FOR 4 SERVINGS)

- Juice of 1 lime
- 225 g silken tofu
- 1 Bird's eye chili
- 2 tbsp. of fresh coriander (chopped)
- 3 avocados

## COOKING DIRECTIONS

1. Combine all ingredients in your blender or food process into a soft chunky mixture.
2. Serve with crudités.

# Waldorf Salad

## INGREDIENTS (FOR 1 SERVINGS)

For Dressing:
- 1 tsp. of Dijon mustard
- 1 tbsp. of Extra virgin olive oil
- Juice of half a lemon
- 1 tsp. of balsamic vinegar

For Salad:
- 10 g lovage or celery leaves (roughly chopped)
- 10 g flat parsley (chopped)
- 50 g walnuts (roughly chopped)
- 100 g apple (roughly chopped)
- 200 g celery (roughly chopped)
- 1 small red onion, roughly chopped
- 1 tbsp. of capers
- 1 head of chicory (chopped)
- 1 small red onion (roughly chopped)

## COOKING DIRECTIONS

1. Mix capers, celery, parsley, apples, onion, walnuts, and lovage in your salad bowl.
2. In another bowl, add your lemon juice, vinegar, mustard, and oil together, and whisk until well combined.
3. Serve dressing over salad.

# Fruit Skewers with Strawberry Dip

## INGREDIENTS (FOR 4 SERVINGS)

- 400 g of strawberries
- 150 g of red grapes
- 1 pineapple (peeled and diced)

## COOKING DIRECTIONS

1. Divide strawberries into 4 places and add to a food processor. Blend until it becomes a smooth paste.
2. Thread grapes, pineapples, and the rest of your strawberries onto a skewer.
3. Serve with strawberry dip.

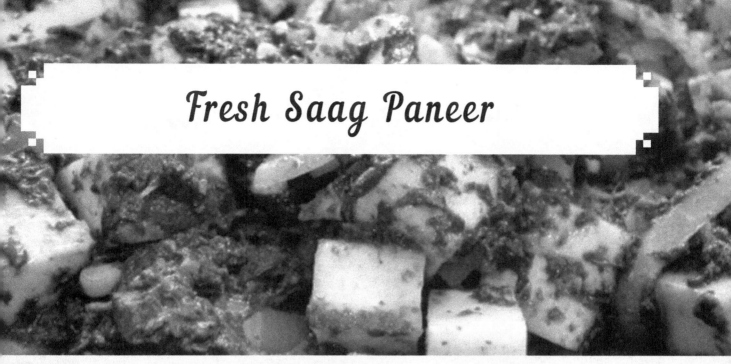

# Fresh Saag Paneer

## INGREDIENTS (FOR 2 SERVINGS)

- 100 g fresh spinach leaves
- 200 g Paneer (cut into cubes)
- 10 g parsley (chopped)
- 10 g coriander (chopped)
- 100 g cherry tomatoes (halved)
- 1/2 tsp. of salt
- Freshly ground black pepper
- 2 tsp. of rapeseed oil
- 1 red onion (chopped)
- 1/2 tsp. of mild chili powder
- 3 cm fresh ginger (peeled and cut into matchsticks)
- 1/4 tsp. of ground turmeric
- 1 clove of garlic (peeled and thinly sliced)
- 1/2 tsp. of ground cumin
- 1 green chili, deseeded and finely sliced
- 1/2 tsp. of ground coriander

## COOKING DIRECTIONS

1. Place a wide lid frying pan over high heat.
2. Add oil to heat up.
3. Season your Paneer with a generous amount of pepper and salt.
4. Sear Paneer in the frying pan until golden brown. Remove with a slotted spoon and set aside.
5. Reduce heat and add onion. Fry for about 5 minutes.
6. Add chili, garlic and ginger. Cook for another 3 minutes.
7. Add tomatoes, cook for 5 minutes.
8. Add salt and spices, stir and add paneer back to the pan. Stir so that the sauce coats the paneer completely.
9. Cover the pan with the lid and let it cook for 5 minutes.
10. Add parsley, spinach and coriander. Stir and cook until spinach wilts.
11. Serve immediately.

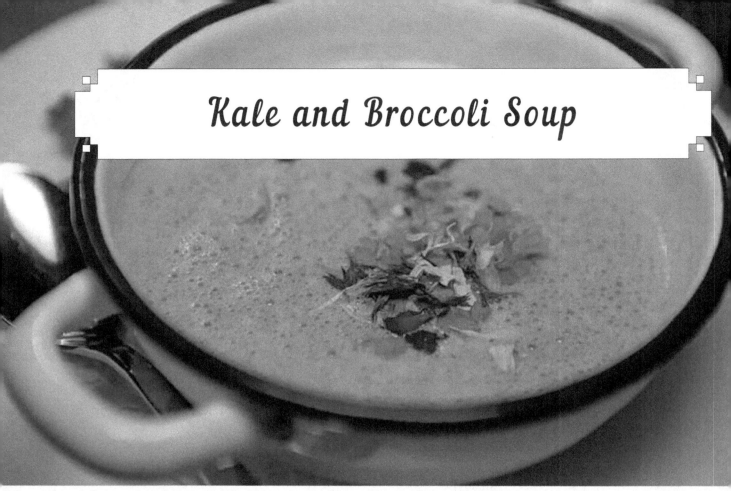

# Kale and Broccoli Soup

## INGREDIENTS (FOR 4 SERVINGS)

- 1 tbsp. of olive oil
- 250 g broccoli
- 300 ml milk
- 250 g kale
- 600 ml vegetable stock
- 1 red onion (chopped)
- 1 potato (peeled and chopped)
- Sea salt and freshly ground black pepper to taste

## COOKING DIRECTIONS

1. Place a saucepan over heat and add olive oil to heat up.
2. Add onions and sauté for 5 minutes.
3. Add broccoli, kale and potato. Stir and cook for 5 minutes.
4. Add milk and vegetable stock. Stir. Let it simmer for 20 minutes.
5. Insert a hand blender into the soup and puree until smooth.
6. Add salt and pepper to taste. Stir.
7. Serve.

# King Prawn Stir-Fry with Buckwheat Noodles

## INGREDIENTS (FOR 1 SERVINGS)

- 5 g celery leaves
- 150 g raw king prawns (shelled, deveined)
- 50 g kale (roughly chopped)
- 75 g soba (buckwheat noodles)
- 20 g red onions (sliced)
- 75 g green beans (chopped)
- 40 g celery (trimmed and sliced)
- 100 ml of chicken stock
- 1 tsp. of fresh ginger (finely chopped)
- 2 tsp. of Extra virgin olive oil
- 2 tsp. of tamari
- 1 Bird's eye chili (finely chopped)
- 1 garlic clove (finely chopped)

## COOKING DIRECTIONS

1. Place a frying pan over high heat and when the oil is hot, add a tsp. of oil and a tsp. of tamari, then add the prawns.
2. Cook the prawns in the pan for 3 minutes. Remove cooked prawns to a platter.
3. Cook noodles according to the instructions on the packet. Drain and set aside.
4. Return the frying pan you used for the chicken back to heat and add your remaining oil to heat up.
5. Add celery, garlic, red onion, chili, beans, and garlic to the pan. Stir and cook for 3 minutes.
6. Add chicken stock, stir, and bring to a boil.
7. Simmer for a minute, and then add celery or lovage.
8. Add the noodles and prawns. Stir and let it boil.
9. Remove from heat and serve.

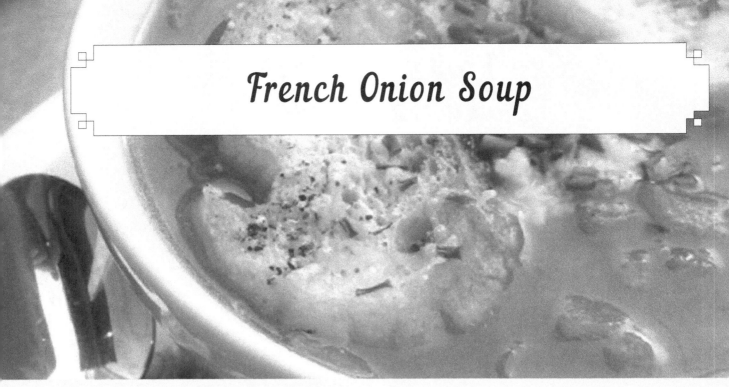

# French Onion Soup

## INGREDIENTS (FOR 4 SERVINGS)

- 1 tbsp. of olive oil
- 750 g red onions (thinly sliced)
- 900 ml beef stock
- 50 g cheddar cheese (shredded)

- 2 slices of wholemeal bread
- 2 tsp. of flour
- 12 g butter

## COOKING DIRECTIONS

1. Place a saucepan over high heat and add butter to melt and heat up.
2. Add onions to the pan and reduce the heat to low. Cook for 25 minutes while stirring continuously.
3. Add flour and stir thoroughly.
4. Add beef stock and stir. Bring to a boil.
5. Reduce heat and allow the soup simmer for 30 minutes.
6. Remove from heat.
7. Sprinkle cheese on the bread slices and grill them until the cheese melts.
8. Serve soup with cheesy bread slices on top.

# Baked Salmon Salad with Creamy Mint Dressing

## INGREDIENTS (FOR 1 SERVINGS)

For Dressing:
- 1 tbsp. of rice vinegar
- 1 tsp. of low-fat mayonnaise
- 2 mint leaves (finely chopped)
- Salt and freshly ground black pepper to taste
- 1 tbsp. of natural yogurt

For Salad:
- 130 g of salmon fillet
- 50 g cucumber (cut into chunks)
- 10 g parsley (roughly chopped)
- 40 g young spinach leaves
- 2 spring onions (trimmed and sliced)
- 40 g mixed salad leaves
- 2 radishes (trimmed and thinly sliced)

## COOKING DIRECTIONS

1. Preheat the oven to 200C/400F.
2. Arrange the salmon fillets on a baking tray with the skin side facing down and bake for 15 to 20 minutes.
3. Remove salmon and set aside.
4. Combine rice wine vinegar, yoghurt, and mayonnaise in a bowl and mix.
5. Season with salt and pepper and mix.
6. Add mint leaves and mix.
7. Let it sit for 5 minutes.
8. Combine salad leaves and spinach in a salad bowl and mix.
9. Add spring onions, radish, parsley, and cucumber to the sides.
10. Flake cooked salmon into the mixture.
11. Drizzle mint dressing over it.
12. Serve.

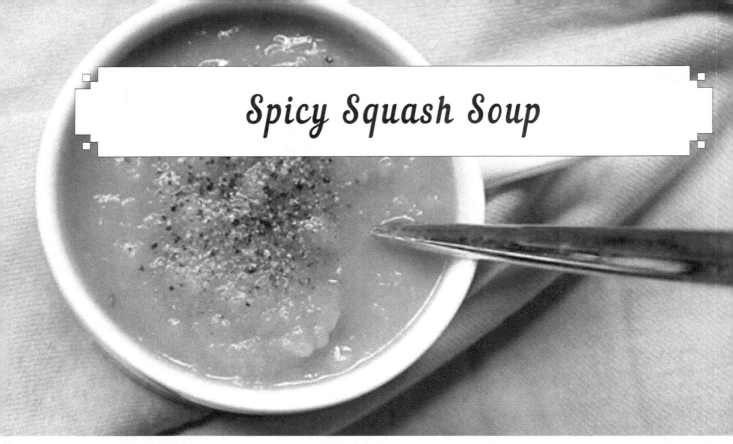

# Spicy Squash Soup

## INGREDIENTS (FOR 4 SERVINGS)

- 2 tbsp. of olive oil
- 150 g of kale
- 600 ml vegetable stock
- 1 butternut squash (peeled, deseeded and chopped)
- 1 tsp. of ground ginger

- 1 red onion (chopped)
- 2 tsp. of turmeric
- 3 Bird's eye chilies (chopped)
- 2 tsp. of turmeric
- 3 cloves of garlic

## COOKING DIRECTIONS

1. Place a saucepan over high heat and add olive oil to heat up.
2. Add onions and butternut squash. Cook for 6 minutes.
3. Add chili, ginger, garlic, turmeric, and kale. Stir and let it cook for 2 minutes.
4. Add vegetable stock and stir. Bring to a boil.
5. Let the soup simmer for 10 minutes.
6. Insert a hand blender into the soup and puree until smooth.
7. Add salt and pepper to taste. Stir.
8. Serve.

# Prawn Arrabbiata

## INGREDIENTS (FOR 1 SERVINGS)

- 400 g canned chopped tomatoes
- 150 g cooked king prawns
- 30 g celery (finely chopped)
- 65 g buckwheat pasta
- 1 tbsp. of Extra virgin olive oil
- 2 tbsp. of white wine
- 1 Bird's eye chili (finely chopped)
- 1 tsp. of dried mixed herbs
- 1 tbsp. of parsley (chopped)

## COOKING DIRECTIONS

1. Place a saucepan over medium heat and add oil to heat up.
2. Add celery, onions, garlic, chili, and dried herbs. Stir and let it cook for 2 minutes.
3. Add wine and stir. Reduce heat and cook for a minute.
4. Add tomatoes, stir, and let it simmer over medium heat for 30 minutes.
5. Add prawns and stir. Cook until prawns turn pink and opaque.
6. Add parsley and stir.
7. Remove from heat.
8. Cook pasta according to instructions on the package.
9. Serve prawn Arrabbiata over pasta.

# Blue Cheese and Celery Soup

## INGREDIENTS (FOR 4 SERVINGS)

- 150 ml single cream
- 125 g blue cheese
- 900 ml of chicken broth
- 25 g butter
- 1 red onion (chopped)
- One 650 g head of celery

## COOKING DIRECTIONS

1. Place a saucepan over high heat and add butter to melt and heat up.
2. Add celery and onion to the pan and cook for 5 minutes or until veggies soften.
3. Add chicken broth and stir. Let it cook for 15 minutes.
4. Add cheese and cream. Stir.
5. Cook until the cheese melts and then serve.

# Coronation Chicken Salad

## INGREDIENTS (FOR 1 SERVINGS)

- 40 g arugula
- 20 g red onion (diced)
- 100 g cooked chicken breast (cut into bite-sized pieces)
- 75 g natural yoghurt
- 1 Bird's eye chili
- 1 Medjool date, finely chopped
- Juice of 1/4 of a lemon
- 6 walnut halves (finely chopped)
- 1/2 tsp. of mild curry powder
- 1 tsp. of ground turmeric
- 1 tsp. of coriander (chopped)

## COOKING DIRECTIONS

1. Combine all your spices with yoghurt, lemon juice, and coriander together in a bowl. Mix well.
2. Add everything else to the bowl and serve over a bed of arugula.

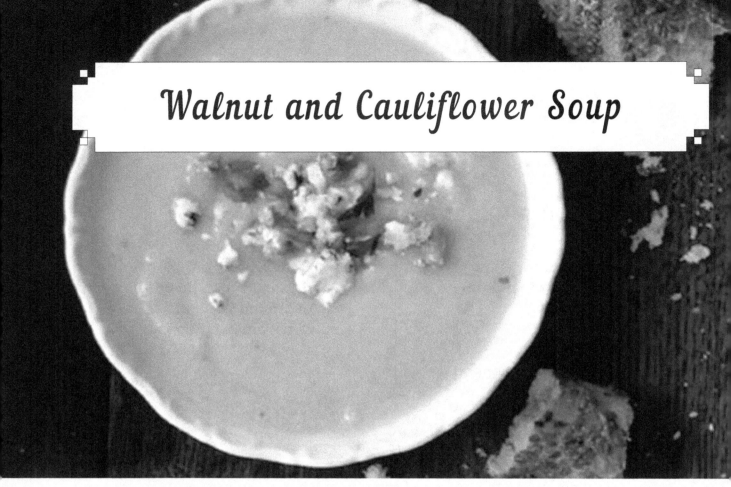

# Walnut and Cauliflower Soup

## INGREDIENTS (FOR 4 SERVINGS)

- 1 tbsp. of olive oil
- 450 g cauliflower (chopped)
- 1/2 tsp. of turmeric
- 100 ml heavy cream
- 900 ml vegetable broth
- 1 red onion (chopped)
- 4 walnuts (chopped in halves)

## COOKING DIRECTIONS

1. Place a saucepan over heat and add olive oil to heat up.
2. Add red onions and cauliflower. Stir continuously for 4 minutes.
3. Add vegetable stock and stir. Bring to a boil.
4. Let the soup simmer for 15 minutes.
5. Add turmeric, double cream and walnuts. Stir and let it cook for 5 minutes.
6. Insert a hand blender into the soup and puree until smooth.
7. Add salt and pepper to taste. Stir.
8. Serve.

# Greek Salad Skewers

## INGREDIENTS (FOR 2 SERVINGS)

For Dressing:
- 1 tsp. of balsamic vinegar
- Handful of oregano (finely chopped)
- Freshly ground black pepper
- Salt to taste
- Handful of basil leaves (finely chopped)
- 1 tbsp. of Extra virgin olive oil
- 1/2 clove garlic (peeled and crushed)
- Juice of 1/2 lemon

For Salad:
- 100 g feta (cut into 8 cubes)
- 100 g cucumber (cut into 4 slices and halved)
- 2 wooden skewers (soaked in water for 30 minutes)
- 1/2 red onion (cut in half and separated into 8 pieces)
- 8 large black olives
- 1 yellow pepper (cut into 8 squares)
- 8 cherry tomatoes

## COOKING DIRECTIONS

1. Soak wooden skewers in water for 30 minutes.
2. Thread the salad ingredients into each skewer in this order: olive, yellow pepper, tomato, red onion, feta, cucumber, olive, yellow pepper, tomato, red onion, feta, and cucumber.
3. Mix all salad dressing ingredients together in a bowl.
4. Pour salad dressing over skewers and serve.

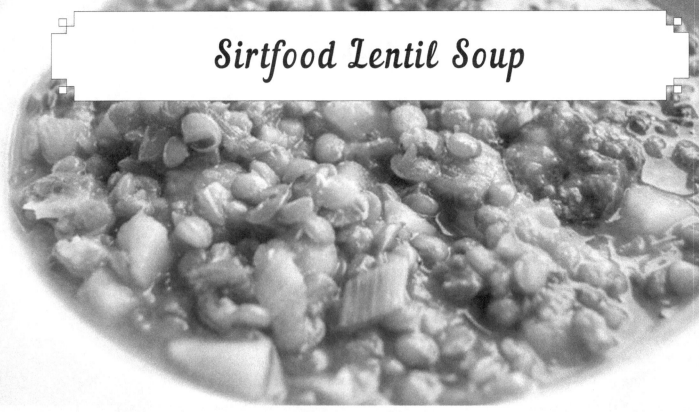

# Sirtfood Lentil Soup

## INGREDIENTS (FOR 4 SERVINGS)

- 1 tsp. of ground coriander
- Sea salt and freshly ground pepper to taste
- 2 tbsp. of olive oil
- 1200 ml vegetable stock
- 175 g red lentils
- 1 tsp. of ground turmeric

- 1 red onion (chopped)
- 1 tsp. of ground cumin
- 1 clove of garlic (chopped)
- 1/2 Bird's eye chili
- 2 carrots (chopped)
- 2 sticks of celery (chopped)

## COOKING DIRECTIONS

1. Place a saucepan over heat and add olive oil to heat up.
2. Add onions and sauté for 5 minutes.
3. Add lentils, coriander, carrots, chili, celery, garlic, turmeric, and cumin. Stir and let it cook for 5 minutes.
4. Add vegetable stock and stir. Bring to a boil.
5. Let the soup simmer for 10 minutes.
6. Insert a hand blender into the soup and puree until smooth.
7. Add salt and pepper to taste. Stir.
8. Serve.

# Sesame Chicken Salad

## INGREDIENTS (FOR 2 SERVINGS)

For Dressing:
- 2 tsp. of soy sauce
- 1 tbsp. of Extra virgin olive oil
- 1 tsp. of clear honey
- Juice of 1 lime
- 1 tsp. of sesame oil

For Salad:
- 150 g cooked chicken (shredded)
- 20 g parsley (chopped)
- 100 g baby kale (roughly chopped)
- 1 tbsp. of sesame seeds
- 60 g pak choi (very finely shredded)
- 1 cucumber (peeled, halved lengthways, deseeded and sliced)
- 1/2 red onion (very finely sliced)

## COOKING DIRECTIONS

1. Place frying pan over heat.
2. When the pan heats up, toast sesame seed in the pan for 2 minutes.
3. Combine honey, olive oil, soy sauce, lime juice, and sesame oil in a bowl and mix together.
4. In another bowl, combine red onion, cucumber, parsley, pak choi, and kale together. Mix well.
5. Serve dressing over salad with shredded chicken on the side and sesame seed sprinkled over it.

# Apple, Kale and Fennel Soup

## INGREDIENTS (FOR 4 SERVINGS)

- 1 tbsp. of olive oil
- 450 g kale (chopped)
- 2 tbsp. of freshly parsley (chopped)
- 200 g fennel (chopped)
- Sea salt and freshly ground black pepper to taste
- 2 apples (peeled, cored and chopped)

## COOKING DIRECTIONS

1. Place a saucepan over heat and add olive oil to heat up.
2. Add fennel and kale to the pan and cook for 5 minutes until fennel softens.
3. Add parsley and apples, stir.
4. Pour hot water in the pan and bring to a boil. Afterwards, let it simmer for 10 minutes.
5. Insert a hand blender into the soup and puree until smooth.
6. Add salt and pepper to taste. Stir.
7. Serve.

# Kale and Feta Salad with Cranberry Dressing

## INGREDIENTS (FOR 1 SERVINGS)

For Cranberry Dressing:
- 3 tbsp. of olive oil
- 75 g of cranberries
- Sea salt
- 2 tsp. of honey
- 1 tbsp. of red wine vinegar
- 3 tbsp. of water
- 1/2 red onion (chopped)

For Salad:
- 4 Medjool dates (chopped)
- 250 g of kale (finely chopped)
- 1 apple (peeled, cored and cubed)
- 75 g of feta cheese
- 50 g walnut (chopped)

## COOKING DIRECTIONS

1. Combine all the salad ingredients into a bowl. Mix.
2. Combine all your dressing ingredients into your blender and process until smooth.
3. Serve dressing over salad.

# Tuna with Lemon Herb Dressing

## INGREDIENTS (FOR 4 SERVINGS)

For Dressing:
- Juice of 1 lemon
- 25 g pitted green olives (chopped)
- 2 tbsp. of olive oil
- 1 tbsp. of fresh basil (chopped)

For Tuna:
- 1 tbsp. of olive oil
- 4 tuna steaks

## COOKING DIRECTIONS

1. Place a griddle pan over heat.
2. Add a tablespoon of olive oil to the pan and let it heat up.
3. Add your tuna steaks to the pan and let it cook for 3 minutes. Flip and cook the other side for another 2 minutes.
4. Combine all dressing ingredients in a mixing bowl and whisk well.
5. Transfer to tuna steaks to a serving platter.
6. Serve dollops of dressing over tuna steaks.
7. Enjoy.

# Tuna, Eggs and Capers Salad

## INGREDIENTS (FOR 1 SERVINGS)

- 100 g cucumber
- 1 red onion (chopped)
- 100 g red or yellow chicory
- 2 tbsp. of fresh parsley
- 150 g canned tuna fish
- 2 tomatoes (chopped)
- 2 eggs (hardboiled and chopped)
- 6 black olives (pitted)
- 25 g arugula leaves
- 2 tbsp. of garlic vinaigrette
- 1 tbsp. of capers

## COOKING DIRECTIONS

1. Combine onion, tuna, tomatoes, olives, cucumber, arugula, parsley, celery, and chicory in a salad bowl and mix.
2. Add garlic vinaigrette into the salad and toss.
3. Serve salad with topped with capers and egg.

# *Sirtfood Chicken Stir-fry*

## INGREDIENTS (FOR 2 SERVINGS)

- 2 tbsp. of soy sauce
- 150 g egg noodles
- 1 clove of garlic
- 50 g cauliflower florets (roughly chopped)
- 1 red bell pepper (chopped)
- 25 g kale (finely chopped)
- 2 chicken breasts
- 25 g mango tout
- 2 stalks of celery (finely chopped)
- 1 tbsp. of olive oil
- 100 ml of chicken stock

## COOKING DIRECTIONS

1. Cook noodles according to the instructions on the package.
2. Make a frying pan over heat and add olive oil to heat up.
3. Add chicken and garlic to the pan. Cook for 5 minutes.
4. Add red bell pepper, mange tout, pepper, kale, cauliflower, and celery. Stir and cook for 4 minutes.
5. Add soy sauce and chicken stock. Stir.
6. Cook for 5 minutes.
7. Add cooked noodles and stir.
8. Serve.

# Nut and Chicory Salad

## INGREDIENTS (FOR 2 SERVINGS)

For Dressing:
- 25 ml of red wine vinegar
- 2 tbsp. of fresh parsley
- 1 tbsp. of olive oil
- 1/2 tsp. of turmeric
- 1/2 tsp. of mustard

For Salad:
- 1 tbsp. of olive oil
- 100 g of green beans
- 2 tomatoes (chopped)
- 100 g of red chicory
- 25 g unsalted peanuts (chopped)
- 100 g of celery (chopped)
- 25 g of walnuts (chopped)
- 25 g of macadamia nuts

## COOKING DIRECTIONS

1. Add all dressing ingredients to a mason jar and shake until well combined.
2. Place a frying pan over medium heat and add a tbsp. of olive oil to heat up.
3. Pour celery, chicory, and green beans into the pan and cook until softened.
4. Add chopped tomatoes and cook for another 2 minutes.
5. Pour everything into a large bowl and pour the dressing in it. Mix everything together.
6. Sprinkle nuts over it.
7. Serve.

# Zucchini Noodles with Mushroom and Lemon Caper Pesto

## INGREDIENTS (FOR 4 SERVINGS)

- 50 g arugula leaves
- 2 tbsp. of lemon capers pesto
- 4 zucchini
- 2 tbsp. of olive oil
- 1 red onion (sliced)
- 10 oyster mushrooms (sliced)

## COOKING DIRECTIONS

1. Spiralize zucchini to form noodles and place them in frying pan over heat and add olive oil.
2. Add onions and mushrooms. Stir and cook until softened.
3. Add pesto and zucchini. Stir.
4. Let it cook for 5 minutes and serve over a bed of arugula.

# Chili Honey Squash

## INGREDIENTS (FOR 4 SERVINGS)

- Juice of 1 lime
- 2 red onions (roughly chopped)
- 1 inch of ginger (peeled and roughly chopped)
- Juice of 1 orange
- 2 cloves of garlic
- 1 tbsp. of olive oil
- 100 ml of vegetable oil
- 1 butternut squash (peeled and chopped)
- 2 Bird's eye chilies (finely chopped)

## COOKING DIRECTIONS

1. Place a pan over heat and add chilies to heat up.
2. Add red onions, ginger, honey, squash, and garlic. Sauté for 3 minutes.
3. Add orange and lime juice. Stir.
4. Add vegetable stock and stir.
5. Let it simmer for 15 minutes and then serve.

# Arugula, Feta, and Strawberry Salad

## INGREDIENTS (FOR 2 SERVINGS)

- 2 tbsp. of flaxseeds
- 75 g of fresh arugula leaves
- 4 walnuts (halved)
- 100 g strawberries (halved)
- 75 g crumbled feta cheese

## COOKING DIRECTIONS

1. Combine all ingredients in a mixing bowl and drizzle with olive oil.
2. Serve.

# Arugula and Serrano Ham

## INGREDIENTS (FOR 4 SERVINGS)

- 2 tbsp. of olive oil
- 175 g of Serrano ham
- 1 tbsp. of orange juice
- 125 g arugula

## COOKING DIRECTIONS

1. Add orange juice and olive oil into a mixing bowl.
2. Add arugula leaves into the mixing bowl and stir so the oil and juice coat the leaves.
3. Serve topped with Serrano Ham.

# Stilton Cheese and Red Chicory Boats

## INGREDIENTS (FOR 4 SERVINGS)

- 1 tbsp. of olive oil
- 200 g of crumbled stilton cheese
- 2 tbsp. of fresh parsley (chopped)
- 200 g red or yellow chicory leaves

## COOKING DIRECTIONS

1. Drizzle chicory leaves with olive oil.
2. Sprinkle cheese on chicory leaves.
3. Grill everything for 4 minutes
4. Sprinkle with parsley.
5. Serve immediately.

# Buckwheat Pasta Salad

## INGREDIENTS (FOR 4 SERVINGS)

- 2 tbsp. of olive oil
- 275 g of buckwheat pasta
- 1/2 of coconut milk
- 225 g of green beans
- 2 tbsp. of smooth peanut butter
- 100 g of cherry tomatoes
- 1 Bird's eye chili (finely chopped)
- 1 red onion (finely chopped)
- 2 cloves of garlic (crushed)
- 1/2 tsp. of turmeric

## COOKING DIRECTIONS

1. First, cook buckwheat pasta according to the instructions on the packet. Drain and set aside.
2. Next, place a frying pan over heat and add olive oil to heat up.
3. Combine coconut milk, peanut butter, chili, tomato puree and turmeric in a bowl and mix together. Set aside.
4. Add onion and garlic and sauté for 1 minute.
5. Add green beans and continue to cook for 3 minutes.
6. Add tomatoes and cook for another 2 minutes.
7. Stir in your cooked buckwheat pasta.
8. Stir in the coconut mixture.
9. Serve.

# Buckwheat and Cheese Cakes

## INGREDIENTS (FOR 2 SERVINGS)

- 1 tbsp. of olive oil
- 100 g of cooked buckwheat (room temperature)
- 2 tbsp. of fresh parsley (chopped)
- 1 large egg
- 2 shallots (chopped)
- 25 g of whole meal breadcrumbs
- 25 g of grated cheddar cheese

## COOKING DIRECTIONS

1. Crack eggs into a mixing bowl and whisk very well.
2. In another bowl, combine parsley, buckwheat, shallot, and cheese. Mix well.
3. Pour whisked eggs into the buckwheat mixture. Mix everything together.
4. Form patties out of the mixture.
5. Pour breadcrumbs into a large tray and spread.
6. Roll patties inside the tray so the breadcrumbs coat the patties.
7. Place a frying pan over heat and add olive oil.
8. Fry patties until golden brown.
9. Serve.

# Tomato, Kale, and Hot Chorizo Salad

## INGREDIENTS (FOR 2 SERVINGS)

- 75 g chorizo Sausage (thinly sliced)
- 225 g kale leaves (finely chopped)
- 2 tbsp. of red wine vinegar
- 2 tbsp. of olive oil
- 1 red onion (finely chopped)

- 2 cloves of garlic
- 8 cherry tomatoes
- Salt and freshly ground black pepper to taste

## COOKING DIRECTIONS

1. Place a frying pan over heat and add olive oil to heat up.
2. Add tomatoes, sliced chorizo, onion, and garlic. Stir.
3. Add kale and red wine vinegar. Cook until kale is soft.
4. Add black pepper and sea salt to taste and serve.

# Braised Celery

## INGREDIENTS (FOR 4 SERVINGS)

- Freshly ground black pepper and sea salt to taste
- 250 g of celery (chopped)
- 25 g butter
- 100ml warm vegetable stock
- 1 tbsp. of fresh parsley (chopped)
- 1 clove of garlic (chopped)
- 1 red onion (chopped)

## COOKING DIRECTIONS

1. Add garlic, vegetable stock, onion and celery to a saucepan placed over heat.
2. Bring to a boil, reduce the heat, and then let it simmer for 10 minutes.
3. Add butter and parsley. Stir.
4. Add pepper and salt to taste and serve.

# Walnut and Red Chicory Slaw

## INGREDIENTS (FOR 4 SERVINGS)

- 2 tbsp. of mayonnaise
- 100 g of red or yellow chicory (shredded)
- 1 red onion (finely chopped)
- 5 stalks of celery (finely chopped)
- 4 walnuts (halved)

## COOKING DIRECTIONS

1. Combine all ingredients in a salad bowl and mix well.
2. Let it sit in the refrigerator for some minutes.
3. Serve.

# Parma and Dates Ham

## INGREDIENTS (FOR 4 SERVINGS)

- 2 slices of Parma ham (cut into strips)
- 12 Medjool dates

## COOKING DIRECTIONS

1. Fold each strip of Parma ham over the dates.
2. Serve.

# Chicory and Smoked Salmon Boats

## INGREDIENTS (FOR 4 SERVINGS)

- 2 tbsp. of olive oil
- 150 g of red or yellow chicory leaves
- Juice of 1 lime
- 150 g of smoked salmon (finely chopped)
- 1/2 red onions (finely chopped)
- 2 tbsp. of fresh parsley (chopped)
- 100 g cucumber (diced)

## COOKING DIRECTIONS

1. Add parsley, salmon, onion, and cucumber to a salad bowl. Mix together.
2. Add lime juice and oil. Toss to combine.
3. Scoop the mixture into the chicory leaves to form chicory boats.
4. Let it sit in the refrigerator for some minutes and then serve.

# Nut and Vegetable Loaf

## INGREDIENTS (FOR 4 SERVINGS)

- 600 ml red wine
- 2 cloves of garlic (chopped)
- 100 ml water
- 2 tbsp. of olive oil
- 4 tbsp. of fresh parsley (chopped)
- 2 tsp. of turmeric powder
- 2 tbsp. of soy sauce
- 1 egg (beaten)

- 175 mushrooms (finely chopped)
- 1 red onion (finely chopped)
- 100 g of haricot beans
- 1 Bird's eye chili
- 100 g of walnuts (finely chopped)
- 2 sticks of celery (finely chopped)
- 100 g of peanuts (finely chopped)

## COOKING DIRECTIONS

1. Preheat your oven to 190C/375F.
2. Combine haricot beans, red wine, nuts, parsley, soy sauce, veggies, eggs and nuts in a bowl. Add water and mix. Set aside.
3. Place a frying pan over heat and add oil to heat up.
4. Add turmeric, garlic, mushrooms, chili, onions, carrots, turmeric and celery. Sauté for 5 minutes.
5. Mix with the haricot beans mixture.
6. Line a large loaf tin with parchment paper.
7. Scoop everything into the loaf tin.
8. Bake for 90 minutes.
9. Let it sit for 10 minutes and then serve.

# Salmon Sirt Super Salad

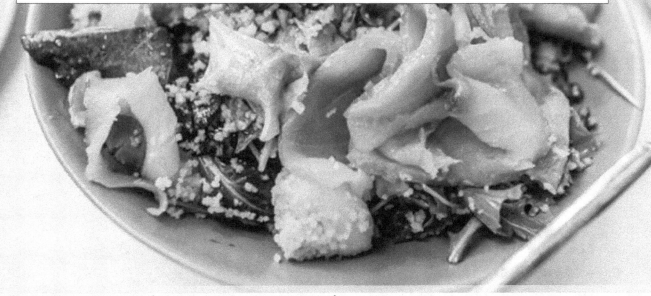

## INGREDIENTS (FOR 1 SERVINGS)

- 10 g celery leaves (chopped)
- 50 g arugula
- 10 g parsley (chopped)
- 15 g walnuts (chopped)
- 50 g chicory leaves
- 100 g smoked salmon slices
- 20 g red onion (sliced)
- 80 g avocado (peeled, stoned and
- sliced)
- 40 g celery (sliced)
- Juice of 1/4 lemon
- 1 tbsp. of capers
- 1 tbsp. of extra-virgin olive oil
- 1 large Medjool date (pitted and chopped)

## COOKING DIRECTIONS

1. Arrange all the leaves on a platter.
2. Combine all other ingredients in a salad bowl and mix.
3. Serve on top of leaves.
4. Enjoy.

# SIRT Muesli

## INGREDIENTS (FOR 2 SERVINGS)

- 100 g plain Greek yoghurt
- 20 g buckwheat flakes
- 10 0g strawberries (hulled and chopped)
- 10 g buckwheat puffs
- 10 g cocoa nibs
- 15 g coconut flakes
- 15g walnuts (chopped)
- 40 g Medjool dates (pitted and chopped)

## COOKING DIRECTIONS

1. Combine all ingredients except strawberries and yogurt in a mixing bowl.
2. Add yogurt and mix.
3. Serve topped with strawberries.

# SIRT Fruit Salad

## INGREDIENTS (FOR 1 SERVINGS)

- 10 blueberries
- 1/2 cup of freshly made green tea
- 10 red seedless grapes
- 1 tsp. of honey
- 1 apple (cored and roughly chopped)
- 1 orange (halved)

## COOKING DIRECTIONS

1. Add honey to the green tea and stir until it dissolves completely.
2. Squeeze out the juice from half of the orange into the glass of green tea. Stir.
3. Place in the refrigerator to cool.
4. Meanwhile, chop the other half of the orange.
5. Remove the drink from refrigerator and add all the fruits inside.

# Dinner Recipes

# Chili Tomato King Prawns

## INGREDIENTS (FOR 4 SERVINGS)

- 2 tbsp. of olive oil
- 100 g pak choi
- 4 tomatoes (chopped)
- 1 tbsp. of fresh parsley (chopped)
- 24 King Prawns (raw, shelled)
- 1 tbsp. of fresh coriander (chopped)
- 2 Bird's eye chilies (chopped)
- For Serving: Cooked Brown rice

## COOKING DIRECTIONS

1. Place a frying pan over high heat and add a tbsp. of oil to heat up.
2. Add prawns to the hot oil and cook until it turns completely pink.
3. Remove prawns and set aside.
4. Add a second tablespoon of oil to the frying pan and add chili peppers, pak choi, and tomatoes. Stir and cook for 3 minutes.
5. Pour the prawns back into the pan and stir.
6. Add coriander and parsley. Stir and remove from heat.
7. Serve over cooked brown rice.

# Turkey Escalope

## INGREDIENTS (FOR 4 SERVINGS)

- 150 g turkey escalope
- 40 g red onion (finely chopped)
- 10 g parsley
- 150 g cauliflower (roughly chopped)
- 30 g sun-dried tomatoes (finely chopped)
- Juice of 1/2 lemon
- 1 Bird's eye chili (finely chopped)
- 1 tbsp. of capers
- 1 tsp. of dried sage
- 2 tsp. of ground turmeric
- 1 clove of garlic (finely chopped)
- 2 tbsp. of Extra virgin olive oil
- 1 tsp. of fresh ginger (finely chopped)

## COOKING DIRECTIONS

1. Pour the cauliflower inside a food processor and pulse for 3 seconds until it looks like couscous. Set aside.
2. Add a tbsp. of oil to a frying pan placed over medium heat, and then add red onion, ginger, chili, and garlic. Fry until soft.
3. Add the cauliflower and turmeric. Continue to cook for about 2 minutes.
4. Add half of your parsley and tomatoes. Stir and cook for 1 minute. Remove from heat and set aside.
5. Now to make your sauce, sprinkle the rest of your oil over the turkey escalope before adding it to the frying pan along with the sage. Fry for each side of the turkey for 3 minutes.
6. Add lemon juice, a tbsp. of water, capers, and the rest of your parsley. Stir.
7. Serve sauce over spiced cauliflower couscous.

# Turkey Curry

## INGREDIENTS (FOR 4 SERVINGS)

- 400 ml full fat coconut milk
- 450 g turkey breasts (chopped)
- 2 red onions (chopped)
- 100 g fresh arugula leaves
- 2 Bird's eye chilies (chopped)
- 2 tbsp. of fresh coriander (finely chopped)
- 5 cloves of garlic (chopped)
- 2 tsp. of turmeric powder
- 3 tsp. of medium curry powder

## COOKING DIRECTIONS

1. Place a saucepan over high heat and add olive oil to heat up.
2. Add red onions and sauté for 5 minutes.
3. Add turkey and garlic and cook for 8 minutes.
4. Add curry powder, turmeric, coriander, chili, and coconut milk. Stir and bring to a boil.
5. Reduce heat and let it simmer for 12 minutes.
6. Serve over cooked brown rice and top with arugula leaves.

# Turmeric Fish with Herbs & Mango Sauce

## INGREDIENTS (FOR 4 SERVINGS)

For Prepping Fish:
- 2 tbsp. of coconut oil
- 1 1/4 lbs. fresh cod fish, boneless and skinless (Chop into 2-inch piece wide and 1/2-inch-thick slices)
- Pinch of sea salt

For Fish Marinade:
- 1 tbsp. of dry sherry
- 1 tbsp. turmeric powder
- 2 tbsp. of olive oil
- 1 tsp. of sea salt
- 2 tsp. of minced ginger
- Mango Dipping Sauce:
- 1 garlic clove
- 1 medium sized ripe mango
- 1 tsp. of dry red chili pepper
- Juice of 1/2 lime
- 2 tbsp. of rice vinegar
- Infused Scallion and Dill Oil:
- 2 cups of fresh dill
- 2 cups scallions (sliced long and thin)
- Pinch of sea salt

Optional Toppings: cashew nuts, pine nuts, lime juice, fresh cilantro

## COOKING DIRECTIONS

1. Marinate the fish in your refrigerator for an hour or overnight, depending on how quickly you want it.
2. Add all the ingredients for your dipping sauce in a blender or food processor, and pulse until smooth or to your desired consistency.
3. Remove your fish from the refrigerator and place a large frying pan over high heat.
4. Add 2 tbsp. of coconut oil to the frying pan to heat up. Reduce heat to medium, and then add the marinated fish to the hot oil.
5. Season the fish with salt. Let it fry for 5 minutes before flipping to the other side. Fry the other side for another 5 minutes or until golden brown.
6. Remove fried fish to a platter.
7. When you remove the fish from the frying pan, reduce the heat and add the rest of your coconut oil to the pan.
8. Add 2 cups of dill and 2 cups of scallion to the oil. Toss gently, and then add a dash of salt.
9. Let it marinate for 30 seconds.
10. Serve infused oil over fried fish with mango dipping sauce on the side.
11. Garnish with nuts, cilantro, and lime.

# Spinach and Cannellini Curry

## INGREDIENTS (FOR 4 SERVINGS)

- 2 tbsp. of olive oil
- 400 g cannellini beans
- 600 ml vegetable stock
- 400 g canned tomatoes
- 1 Bird's eye chili (finely chopped)
- 150 g cauliflower florets
- 1 tsp. of curry powder
- 75 g spinach
- 1 1/2 tsp. of turmeric
- 1 red onion (chopped)
- 1 tsp. of ground cumin
- 3 cloves of garlic (chopped)
- 1 carrot (chopped)
- For Serving: Cooked Brown rice

## COOKING DIRECTIONS

1. Place a saucepan over high heat and add oil to heat up.
2. Add garlic, onions, carrots, and cauliflower, sauté for 5 minutes.
3. Add curry powder, cumin, chili and turmeric, and let it cook for another 2 minutes.
4. Add the stock and stir.
5. Add cannellini beans and tomatoes, stir and bring to a boil.
6. Reduce heat and let it simmer for 30 minutes.
7. Add spinach and cook for another 2 minutes.
8. Serve over brown rice

# Chargrilled Beef with Onion Rings, Garlic, Kale and Herb Roasted Potatoes

## INGREDIENTS (FOR 2 SERVINGS)

- 50 g beef fillet steak (3.5 cm-thick)
- 50 g kale (sliced)
- 100 g potatoes (peeled and cut into 2cm dice)
- 5 g parsley (finely chopped)
- 1 tbsp. Extra virgin olive oil
- 50 g red onion (cut into rings)
- 1 tsp. of corn flour
- 1 garlic clove (finely chopped)
- 40 ml red wine
- 1 tsp. of tomato purée
- 150 ml beef stock

## COOKING DIRECTIONS

1. Dissolve corn flour in 1 tbsp. of water.
2. Pre-heat your oven to 220C/240F.
3. Place a saucepan over high heat and add water to boil.
4. When the water starts to boil, add your potatoes and reduce the heat to medium. Let the potatoes cook for 5 minutes.
5. Drain the potatoes.
6. Add a tsp. of oil to a roasting tin and put the potatoes in the roasting tin. Roast in your oven for 40 minutes. Flip every 10 minutes.
7. Remove from oven and sprinkle with parsley. Stir and set aside.
8. Steam kale for 3 minutes, drain and set aside.
9. Add a tsp. of oil to a pan placed over heat add onions and fry for 5 minutes or until caramelized. Set aside.
10. Add garlic to half a tsp. of oil. Fry for a minute.
11. Add steamed kale, stir and cook for 2 minutes. Set aside and keep warm.
12. Place an oven-proof frying pan over high heat.
13. When the pan starts to smoke, add half a tsp. of oil, and then add your meat. Sear in the hot pan until the meat is cooked to your desired taste.
14. Remove pan from heat and place in your oven to cook according to prescribed cooking times.
15. Remove pan from oven, remove meat from pan, then set aside to rest.
16. Pour wine into the pan and scrape the sides and bottoms of the pan to free up any meat residue.
17. Place pan over heat and cook until wine becomes thick like syrup.
18. Add tomato puree and stock. Stir and bring to a boil.
19. Add corn flour paste and stir. Cook for 5 minutes.
20. Serve steak with red wine sauce, roasted potatoes, caramelized onions rings, and kale on the side.

# Roast Leg of Lamb with Red Wine Sauce

## INGREDIENTS (FOR 6 SERVINGS)

- 300 ml red wine
- 1.5 kg leg of lamb
- 1/2 tsp. of sea salt
- 5 cloves of garlic
- 1 tbsp. of olive oil
- 6 sprigs of rosemary
- 1 tbsp. of honey
- 3 tbsp. of parsley

## COOKING DIRECTIONS

1. Pour the parsley, rosemary, salt, and garlic inside your blender and process into a smooth paste.
2. Place lamb meat on a tray and use a knife to make small incisions all over the lamb and rub the herb paste into each incision.
3. Use your hands to massage so the mixture can penetrate the meat.
4. Drizzle all the oil over the meat.
5. Use foil paper to cover it.
6. Place in the oven and let it cook for 1 hour 30 minutes.
7. While the meat is cooking, place a small saucepan over high heat and add honey to melt.
8. Add red wine and stir.
9. Reduce the heat and let it simmer for 5 minutes.
10. Bring the lamb out of the oven and pour the red wine sauce all over it.
11. Return it to the oven and cook for another 6 minutes.
12. Serve.

# Sirt Chili Con Carne

## INGREDIENTS (FOR 4 SERVINGS)

- 150 g canned kidney beans
- 160 g buckwheat
- 400 g lean minced beef
- 2 x 400g tins chopped tomatoes
- 5 g parsley (chopped)
- 5 g coriander (chopped)
- 1 red onion (finely chopped)
- 300 ml beef stock
- 3 garlic cloves (finely chopped)
- 1 tbsp. of cocoa powder
- 2 Bird's eye chilies (finely chopped)
- 1 tbsp. of tomato purée
- 1 tbsp. of Extra virgin olive oil
- 1 red pepper (cored, seeds removed and cut into bite-sized pieces)
- 1 tbsp. of ground cumin
- 150ml red wine
- 1 tbsp. of ground turmeric

## COOKING DIRECTIONS

1. Place a non-stick frying pan over medium heat. Add oil to heat up.
2. Add garlic, onion, and chili to the pan. Fry for 3 minutes.
3. Increase heat to high and add minced beef. Cook until beef is browned on all sides.
4. Add red wine and scrape the sides and bottom of the pan to free up all stuck meat residue. Leave to cook until the liquid is reduced by half.
5. Add tomatoes, kidney beans, tomato puree, red pepper and beef stock. Stir.
6. Let it simmer for one hour.
7. Add chopped herbs, stir, and then remove from heat.
8. Cook buckwheat according to instructions on the pack.
9. Serve with buckwheat.

# Steak and Mushroom Noodles

## INGREDIENTS (FOR 4 SERVINGS)

- 2 tbsp. of olive oil
- 100 g of shiitake mushrooms (halved)
- 1 L warm water
- 100 g chestnut mushrooms (sliced)
- 1 tbsp. of fresh coriander (chopped)
- 150 g Udon noodles
- 1-inch piece of fresh ginger (finely chopped)
- 75 g of kale (finely chopped)
- 2 sirloin steaks
- 75 g of baby leaf spinach (chopped)
- 2 tbsp. of miso paste
- 1 star anise
- 1 red onion (finely chopped)
- 1 red chili (finely sliced)

## COOKING DIRECTIONS

1. Place a saucepan over high heat and add water.
2. Add star anise, ginger, and miso. Stir and bring to a boil.
3. Reduce heat to low and allow it to simmer for 10 minutes.
4. In another pot, cook your noodles according to the instructions on the package.
5. Cook steak in a separate saucepan and cook for 3 minutes. Flip and cook the other side for 2 minutes.
6. Remove meat and set aside.
7. Add mushrooms, coriander, spinach, and kale to the miso soup and let it cook for 5 minutes.
8. Place a separate pan over heat and add the remaining oil.
9. Add onions and chili and fry for 4 minutes or until onions are soft.
10. Serve noodles with miso soup and top with sliced steaks and veggies on the side.

# Chickpea, Quinoa and Turmeric Curry

## INGREDIENTS (FOR 6 SERVINGS)

- 400 g canned chopped tomatoes
- 500 g new potatoes (halved)
- 150 g spinach
- 400 g can of coconut milk
- 400 g can of chickpeas (drained and rinsed)
- 180 g quinoa

- 3 garlic cloves, crushed
- Salt and pepper
- 3 tsp. ground turmeric
- 1 tbsp. of tomato purée
- 1 tsp. ground coriander
- 1 tsp. ground ginger
- 1 tsp. chili powder

## COOKING DIRECTIONS

1. Pour cold water in a large pot and add the potatoes to the pot. Let the water cover the potatoes just a little bit.
2. Cook potatoes for 25 minutes then drain.
3. Now, place a saucepan pan over medium heat and add the drained potatoes, coriander, garlic, ginger, turmeric, coconut milk, tomatoes and tomato puree. Stir and bring everything to a boil.
4. Add pepper and salt. Stir.
5. Add a cup of water and quinoa. Stir and reduce heat to low.
6. Place a lid over the saucepan and allow it to simmer for 15 minutes while stirring occasionally.
7. Add chickpea, stir, and cook for another 10 minutes.
8. Add spinach, stir, and cook for 5 more minutes.
9. Confirm that quinoa is crunchy but well cooked.
10. Serve.

# Spicy Cod Fillets

## INGREDIENTS (FOR 4 SERVINGS)

- 4 tbsp. of olive oil
- 4 150 g cod fillets
- 2 cloves of garlic (chopped)
- 2 Bird's eye chilies
- 2 tbsp. of fresh parsley

## COOKING DIRECTIONS

1. Place a pan over medium heat and add olive oil to heat up.
2. Add cod fillets to the hot oil and cook one aide for 4 minutes. Flip and cook the other side for another 4 minutes.
3. Remove fish and set aside. Keep it warm.
4. Add the rest of your olive oil to the pan and add chopped garlic, chili, and parsley. Stir.
5. Serve fish and serve warm chili and garlic sauce over it.

# Turmeric Chicken & Kale Salad with Honey Lime Dressing

## INGREDIENTS (FOR 2 SERVINGS)

**For Dressing:**
- 1/2 tsp. sea salt
- 1/2 tsp. of pepper
- 3 tbsp. of lime juice
- 1/2 tsp. of Dijon mustard
- 1 small garlic clove (finely diced)
- 1 tsp. raw honey
- 3 tbsp. of Extra virgin olive oil

**For the Salad:**
- 1/2 avocado (sliced)
- 2 cups of broccoli florets
- Handful of fresh coriander leaves (chopped)
- 2 tbsp. pumpkin seeds (pepitas)
- Handful of fresh parsley leaves (chopped)
- 3 large kale leaves (stems removed and chopped)

**For Chicken:**
- 300 g chickens mince
- 1 tbsp. of coconut oil
- 1/2 tsp. of salt
- 1/2 tsp. of pepper
- 1/2 medium brown onion (diced)
- Juice of 1/2 lime
- 1 large garlic clove (finely diced)
- 1 tsp. lime zest
- 1 tsp. turmeric powder

## COOKING DIRECTIONS

1. Place a small frying pan over medium heat and add coconut oil to heat up.
2. Sauté onions in the oil for 5 minutes.
3. Add garlic and stir.
4. Add chicken mince, stir, and cook for 3 minutes while stirring occasionally.
5. Add pepper, turmeric, lime juice, salt and lime zest. Stir.
6. Allow it cook for 4 minutes before removing from heat. Set aside.
7. Place a small saucepan over heat and add 2 cups of water.
8. Bring water to a boil then add broccoli florets. Let it cook for 2 minutes.
9. Rinse cooked broccoli over cold water and cut each floret into 4 pieces.
10. Toast the pumpkin seeds in a frying pan for 2 minutes. Season with salt and set aside.
11. Add all dressing ingredients to a blender and pulse until smooth.
12. Add chopped kale leaves to a salad bowl and pour dressing over it. Use your hands to massage the dressing into the kale leaves.
13. Add cooked chicken with the sauce to the bowl and stir.
14. Add toasted pumpkin seeds, broccolini, avocado slices, and fresh herbs mix everything together and serve.

# Tender Spiced Lamb

## INGREDIENTS (FOR 8 SERVINGS)

- 2 tbsp. of olive oil
- 1.35 kg lamb shoulder
- 1/4 tsp. of ground cinnamon
- 3 red onions (sliced)
- 1/2 tsp. of ground coriander
- 1 tsp. ground cumin
- 1 Bird's eye chili (finely chopped)
- 3 cloves of garlic (crushed)
- 1 tsp. of turmeric
- For Serving: Couscous

## COOKING DIRECTIONS

1. Combine garlic, chili, a tbsp. of olive oil, and your spices in a bowl and whisk together.
2. Add the lamb to the spice mixture and mix so that the mixture coats the lamb meat. Let it sit for an hour.
3. Preheat your oven to 170C/325F.
4. Place a saucepan over heat and add 1 tablespoon of oil to heat up.
5. Add the lamb to the pan and brown on all sides for 4 minutes.
6. Transfer everything into an ovenproof dish and add red onions.
7. Cover the dish with foil paper and bake in your oven for 4 hours.
8. Serve over couscous.

# Buckwheat Noodles with Chicken Kale & Miso Dressing

## INGREDIENTS (FOR 2 SERVINGS)

For Noodles:
- 150 g of buckwheat noodles
- 1 medium free-range chicken breast (diced)
- 3 handfuls of kale leaves (removed from the stem and roughly cut)
- 3 tbsp. of Tamari sauce
- 4 shiitake mushrooms (sliced)
- 2 large garlic cloves (finely diced)
- 1 tsp. of coconut oil
- 1 long red chili (thinly sliced)
- 1 brown onion (finely diced)

For Dressing:
- 1 tbsp. of extra-virgin olive oil
- 1 tsp. of sesame oil
- 1 1/2 tbsp. of fresh organic miso
- 1 tbsp. of lemon
- 1 tbsp. of Tamari sauce

## COOKING DIRECTIONS

1. Place a medium saucepan over high heat and add 2 cups of water. Bring to a boil.
2. Add kale to the boiling water and let it cook until slightly wilted.
3. Remove kale from the water and set aside.
4. Bring the water back to a boil and add soba noodles. Cook for 5 minutes. Rinse under cold water and set aside too.
5. Place a clean saucepan over high heat and add a tsp. of coconut oil to heat up.
6. Fry shiitake mushrooms in the pan for one and half minutes on each side.
7. Add chili and onions and sauté for 3 minutes.
8. Add chicken, stir, and continue to cook for 5 minutes.
9. Add tamari sauce, garlic, and a splash of water. Stir and continue to cook for 3 minutes.
10. Check to ensure that the chicken is well cooked, and then add the kale and soba noodles. Stir.
11. Add all ingredients for miso dressing in a Mason jar and shake to combine.
12. Serve miso dressing over buckwheat noodles and chicken.

# Sirtfood Thai Tofu Curry

## INGREDIENTS (FOR 4 SERVINGS)

- 1 inner stalk of lemon grass
- 400 g tofu (diced)
- 2 tbsp. of tomato puree
- 200 g sugar snap peas
- 2 Bird's eye chilies
- 2 cloves of garlic (chopped)
- 2-inch piece of fresh ginger (chopped)
- 2 red onions (chopped)

- Juice of 1 lime
- 1 tbsp. of fresh coriander (chopped)
- 1 tbsp. of olive oil
- 1 tsp. of cumin
- 200 ml vegetable stock
- 300 ml of coconut milk
- For Serving: Cooked brown rice

## COOKING DIRECTIONS

1. Place a frying pan over high heat and add olive oil to heat up.
2. Add onions and sauté for 4 minutes.
3. Add garlic, chili, ginger cumin, and sauté for another 3 minutes.
4. Add lemongrass, tomato puree, lime juice, sugar snap peas, and tofu. Stir and let it cook for 3 more minutes.
5. Add vegetable stock, coriander, and coconut milk. Stir and let it simmer for 5 minutes.
6. Serve over cooked brown rice with a handful of arugula leaves on the side.

# Fragrant Asian Hotpot

## INGREDIENTS (FOR 2 SERVINGS)

- 20 g sushi ginger (chopped)
- 10 g parsley stalks (finely chopped)
- 50 g cooked water chestnuts (drained)
- 10 g coriander stalks (finely chopped)
- 50 g rice noodles (cooked according to packet instructions)
- 5 0g broccoli (cut into small florets)
- 100 g firm tofu (chopped)
- 50 g beansprouts
- 1 tbsp. of good-quality miso paste
- 100 g raw tiger prawns
- 1 tsp. of tomato purée
- 1/2 carrot (peeled and cut into matchsticks)
- 1 star anise (crushed)
- 500ml chicken stock
- Juice of 1/2 lime

## COOKING DIRECTIONS

1. Place a large saucepan over high heat.
2. Pour the chicken stock inside the pan.
3. Add coriander stalks, tomato puree, parsley stalks lime juice, and star anise. Stir.
4. Cover the saucepan and let it simmer for 10 minutes.
5. Add water chestnuts, carrot, prawns, tofu, noodles, and broccolini. Stir and cook until the prawns are done.
6. Add miso paste and sushi ginger. Stir and remove from heat immediately.
7. Garnish with coriander leaves and parsley.
8. Serve.

# Goat Cheese and Tomato Pizza

## INGREDIENTS (FOR 2 SERVINGS)

For Topping:
- 75 g of tomato paste
- 75 g feta cheese (crumbled)

For Pizza:
- Pinch of salt
- 1 tsp. of olive oil
- 225 g buckwheat flour
- 150 ml water
- 2 tsp. of dried yeast

## COOKING DIRECTIONS

1. Combine all ingredients for the pizza into a bowl and mix together. Let it sit for 1 hour.
2. Roll the dough to a preferred size.
3. Spoon the tomato pasta on to the bottom of the pizza dough and add toppings to the top.
4. Bake for 20 minutes.
5. Serve.

# Lamb, Butternut Squash and Date Tagine

## INGREDIENTS (FOR 4 SERVINGS)

- 400 g canned chickpeas (drained)
- 800 g lamb neck fillet (cut into 2cm chunks)
- 500 g butternut squash (chopped into 1cm cubes)
- 100 g Medjool dates (pitted and chopped)
- 400 g canned chopped tomatoes, plus half a can of water
- 2 tbsp. olive oil
- 1/2 tsp. salt
- 1 red onion (sliced)
- 2 tsp. ground turmeric
- 2 cm ginger (grated)
- 1 cinnamon stick
- 3 garlic cloves (grated)
- 2 tsp. cumin seeds
- 1 tsp. chili flakes (or to taste)
- For Serving: Cooked rice

## COOKING DIRECTIONS

1. Pre-heat your oven to 140C/280F.
2. Coat a large ovenproof saucepan with 2 tablespoons of olive oil.
3. Place the saucepan over medium heat and add sliced onions. Cook onions for 5 minutes or until soft (not brown).
4. Add ginger, grated garlic, cinnamon, turmeric, cumin, and chili. Stir and let it cook for a minute.
5. Add a splash of water and stir.
6. Add lamb chunks and stir to allow the sauce to coat the meat and season with salt and stir.
7. Add tomatoes and chopped dates. Stir.
8. Add a cup of water and stir and bring to a boil.
9. Remove from heat, place on your oven, and cook for 45 minutes.
10. Add butternut squash and cook for another 30 minutes.
11. Remove from oven and add chopped coriander.
12. Serve with cooked rice.

# Roasted Balsamic Veggies

## INGREDIENTS (FOR 4 SERVINGS)

- 4 fresh tomatoes (chopped)
- Sea salt and freshly ground black pepper
- 1 tsp. of mustard
- 2 red onions (chopped)
- 2 tbsp. of balsamic vinegar
- 3 sweet potatoes (peeled and chopped)
- 3 tbsp. of olive oil
- 100 g of red chicory
- 2 tbsp. of fresh parsley (chopped
- 1 Bird's eye chili (deseeded and chopped)
- 300 g of potatoes (peeled and chopped)
- 100 g of kale (finely chopped)
- 5 stalks of celery (chopped)
- 2 tbsp. of fresh coriander

## COOKING DIRECTIONS

1. Pre-heat your oven to 200C/400 F.
2. In a mixing bowl combine coriander, olive oil, parsley, mustard, and balsamic vinegar. Mix everything together well.
3. Add every other ingredient into the mixing bowl and season with salt and pepper. Toss to coat.
4. Transfer everything into an ovenproof dish and bake in the oven for 45 minutes.
5. Serve.

# Turmeric Baked Salmon

## INGREDIENTS (FOR 1 SERVINGS)

- 150 g salmon (skinned)
- 130 g tomato (cut into 8 wedges)
- 150 g celery (cut into 2cm lengths)
- 60 g canned green lentils
- 40 g red onion (finely chopped)
- 100 ml chicken/vegetable stock
- 1 tsp. of Extra virgin olive oil
- 1 tsp. of mild curry powder
- 1 tsp. of Ground turmeric
- 1 Bird's eye chili (finely chopped)
- Juice of 1/4 lemon
- 1 cm fresh ginger (finely chopped)
- 1 garlic clove (finely chopped)
- 1 tbsp. of parsley (chopped)
- 1 tsp. of Extra virgin olive oil

## COOKING DIRECTIONS

1. Pre-heat your oven to 200C/400F.
2. Place a frying pan over medium-low heat and add olive oil to heat up.
3. Add celery, garlic, ginger, chili, and onions. Fry for 2 minutes.
4. Add curry powder and cook for 1 minute.
5. Add tomato, lentils, and stock. Stir and let it simmer for 10 minutes.
6. Add parsley and stir.
7. Place Salmon on a tray and rub a mixture of oil, lemon juice, and turmeric all over it.
8. Bake in the oven for 10 minutes.
9. Serve spicy celery sauce with baked salmon.

# Mussels in Red Wine Sauce

## INGREDIENTS (FOR 2 SERVINGS)

- Juice of 1 lemon
- 800 g mussels
- 400 ml red wine
- 2x400 g canned chopped tomatoes
- 4 cloves of garlic (crushed)
- 25 g of butter
- 4 cloves of garlic (crushed)
- 1 Bird's eye chili (finely chopped)
- 1 tbsp. of fresh parsley (chopped)
- 1 tbsp. of fresh chives (chopped)

## COOKING DIRECTIONS

1. Wash mussels and remove their beards.
2. Place a large saucepan over heat and add butter to melt.
3. Add red wine and stir.
4. Reduce the heat to low and add garlic, parsley, chili, and chives. Stir continuously as you add.
5. Now add the mussels with lemon juice and tomatoes. Stir and cover the pan. Allow it to cook for 3 minutes.
6. Remove from heat and take out any mussels that didn't open up and discard them.
7. Serve.

# Baked Potatoes with Spicy Chickpea Stew

## INGREDIENTS (FOR 4 SERVINGS)

- 2 x 400g canned chickpeas (with water)
- 2 x 400g canned chopped tomatoes
- 4 baking potatoes (pricked all over)
- Salt and pepper to taste
- 2 tbsp. olive oil
- 2 tbsp. parsley
- 2 red onions, finely chopped
- 2 yellow peppers (chopped into bite-sized pieces)
- 4 cloves garlic (crushed)
- 2 tbsp. of unsweetened cocoa powder
- 2 cm ginger (grated)
- Splash of water
- 2 tsp. of chili flakes
- 2 tbsp. of turmeric
- 2 tbsp. of cumin seeds

## COOKING DIRECTIONS

1. Pre-heat your oven to 200C/400 F.
2. Arrange your potatoes on a baking tray and place it in the oven to cook for an hour.
3. Place a wide sauce pan over heat and add olive oil to heat up.
4. Add chopped red onion and sauté for 5 minutes.
5. Add garlic, chili, cumin, and ginger stir and reduce the heat to low. Cook for 10 minutes.
6. Add a splash of water and turmeric. Stir and cook for another minute.
7. Add cocoa powder, tomatoes, chickpeas, and yellow pepper. Stir and bring to a boil.
8. Reduce the heat and let it cook for 45 minutes.
9. Add 2 tbsp. of parsley, and season with salt and pepper.
10. Serve sauce over baked potatoes.

# Beans and Chicken Casserole

## INGREDIENTS (FOR 4 SERVINGS)

- 2 red onions (chopped)
- 1 tbsp. of olive oil
- 1 clove of garlic
- 400 g tomatoes (chopped)
- 2 red bell peppers
- 400 g canned cannellini beans
- 4 large mushrooms

- 8 chicken thighs (skinned)
- 4 sticks of celery
- 2 carrots (peeled and finely chopped)
- 1.75 liters of chicken stock
- 2 tbsp. of soy sauce
- For Serving: **Boiled New Potatoes**

## COOKING DIRECTIONS

1. Place a saucepan over heat and add olive oil to heat up.
2. Add onions and garlic, and sauté for 5 minutes.
3. Add chicken and cook for another 6 minutes.
4. Add cannellini beans, mushrooms, carrots, red bell pepper, celery and stir.
5. Add tomatoes, soy sauce and chicken broth. Stir and bring to a boil.
6. Allow it simmer for 45 minutes.
7. Serve over boiled new potatoes.

# Kale and Red Onion Dhal with Buckwheat

## INGREDIENTS (FOR 4 SERVINGS)

- 160 g buckwheat
- 160 g red lentils
- 100 g kale
- 1 tbsp. of olive oil
- 200 ml water
- 1 small red onion (sliced)
- 400 ml coconut milk

- 3 garlic cloves (crushed)
- 2 tsp. garam masala
- 2 cm ginger (grated)
- 2 tsp. turmeric
- 1 Bird's eye chili (deseeded and finely chopped)

## COOKING DIRECTIONS

1. Place a deep saucepan over heat and add olive oil to heat up.
2. Add sliced onions, stir, and cook for 5 minutes.
3. Add chili, ginger, and garlic. Stir and cook for 1 minute more.
4. Add a cup of water, coconut milk and red lentils. Stir and let it cook for 20 minutes.
5. Add kale and let it cook for 5 minutes.
6. Cook buckwheat for 15 minutes and drain.
7. Serve over buckwheat.

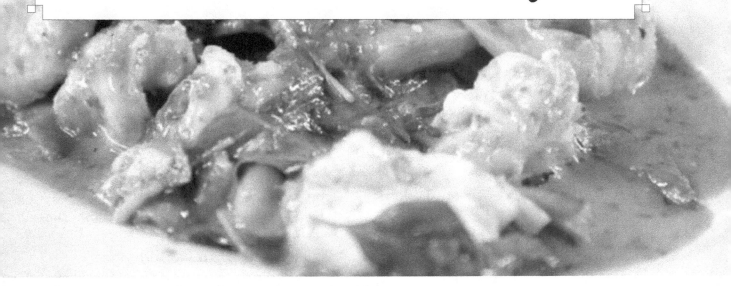

# Coconut and Prawn Curry

## INGREDIENTS (FOR 4 SERVINGS)

- Juice of 1 lime
- 400 g of canned and chopped tomatoes)
- 1 tbsp. of olive oil
- 400 g of large prawns (shelled and raw)
- 400 ml of coconut milk
- 25 g fresh coriander (finely chopped)
- 1/2 tsp. of turmeric
- 3 red onions (finely chopped)
- 1/2 tsp. of ground coriander
- 2 Bird's eye chilies
- 3 cloves of garlic (crushed)
- For Serving: Cooked Rice

## COOKING DIRECTIONS

1. Pour lime juice into a blender and add half of your coriander, onions, chilies, tomatoes, turmeric, and garlic. Pulse until smooth.
2. Place a frying pan over heat and add olive oil to heat up.
3. Pour your blended paste into the pan and fry for 3 minutes.
4. Add coconut milk and stir.
5. Add prawns and cook until it turns pinkish.
6. Add fresh coriander and stir.
7. Serve over cooked rice.

# Kale, Edamame and Tofu Curry

## INGREDIENTS (FOR 4 SERVINGS)

- 200 g kale leaves (stalks removed and torn)
- 200 g firm tofu (chopped into cubes)
- 250 g dried red lentils
- 50 g frozen soya edamame beans
- Juice of 1 lime
- 1 tbsp. of rapeseed oil
- 2 tomatoes (roughly chopped)
- 1 large onion (chopped)
- 1 liter boiling water
- 4 cloves garlic (peeled and grated)
- 1 tsp. of salt
- A 7 cm piece of fresh ginger (peeled and grated)
- 1/2 tsp. of ground cumin
- 1 red chili (deseeded and thinly sliced)
- 1 tsp. of paprika
- 1/2 tsp. of ground turmeric
- 1 red chili, deseeded and thinly sliced

## COOKING DIRECTIONS

1. Place a heavy-bottomed pan over low heat.
2. Add oil to the pan to heat up.
3. Add onion to the pan and sauté for 5 minutes.
4. Add chili, ginger, and garlic. Stir and sauté for 2 minutes.
5. Add turmeric, salt, paprika, cumin and cayenne. Stir.
6. Add red lentils. Stir.
7. Let it simmer for 10 minutes, then reduce the heat and allow it to cook for another 20 minutes until it forms a porridge-like consistency.
8. Add tofu, soya beans and tomatoes. Stir and let it cook for 5 minutes.
9. Add curry leaves and ginger. Stir and cook until kale is tender and serve.

# Sirtfood Moroccan Chicken Casserole

## INGREDIENTS (FOR 4 SERVINGS)

- 2 tbsp. of fresh coriander
- 1 Bird's eye chili (chopped)
- 60 ml water
- 25 g corn flour
- 250 g canned chickpeas
- 600 ml chicken stock
- 1 tsp. of ground turmeric
- 1 tsp. of ground cinnamon
- 1 tsp. of ground cumin
- 4 chicken breasts (cubed)
- 1 carrot (chopped)
- 4 Medjool dates (halved)
- 1 red onion (sliced)
- 6 dried apricots (halved)
- For Serving: Cooked Buckwheat Pasta

## COOKING DIRECTIONS

1. Place a large saucepan over high heat and add chicken stock.
2. Add chickpeas, chicken, turmeric, cumin, carrots, turmeric, chili and cinnamon. Stir and bring to a boil.
3. Reduce heat to low.
4. Add apricots and dated. Stir and allow simmer for 10 minutes.
5. Mix corn flour with water to form a paste.
6. Pour it into the pan and mix.  Continue to cook until thickens.
7. Add cilantro and stir.
8. Serve over cooked buckwheat pasta.

# Aromatic Chicken Breast with Kale, Red Onion, and Salsa

## INGREDIENTS (FOR 2 SERVINGS)

- 50 g buckwheat
- 120 g skinless, boneless chicken breast
- 20 g red onion (sliced)
- 50 g kale (chopped)

- 2 tsp. of ground turmeric
- 1 tsp. of fresh ginger (chopped)
- Juice of 1/4 lemon
- 1 tbsp. of Extra virgin olive oil

## COOKING DIRECTIONS

1. Pre-heat your oven to 220C/240F.
2. Remove the seeds from the tomato and chop it finely. Save the tomato juice as you chop.
3. Pour chopped tomatoes in a bowl and add lemon juice, chili, parsley and capers. Mix. Set salsa aside.
4. Place the chicken breast in a bowl and add lemon juice, a tsp. of turmeric, and some oil.
5. Let it marinate for 10 minutes.
6. Please an ovenproof frying pan over high heat and add the chicken cook until browned on every side.
7. Remove the frying pan from heat and bake in the oven for 10 minutes.
8. Steam kale for 5 minutes
9. Fry ginger and red onions in hot oil until soft, then add steamed kale and stir. Cook for a minute. Set aside.
10. Cook buckwheat pasta according to instructions and the package.
11. Serve buckwheat pasta with salsa, vegetables, and chicken.

# Salmon and Capers

## INGREDIENTS (FOR 4 SERVINGS)

- Zest of 1 lemon
- 75 g of Greek Yogurt
- 2 tsp. of fresh parsley
- 4 salmon fillets (without skin)
- 1 tbsp. of capers (chopped)
- 4 tsp. of Dijon mustard
- For Serving: Green leafy salad

## COOKING DIRECTIONS

1. Pour yogurt in a mixing bowl and add lemon zest, mustard, capers and parsley. Mix well.
2. Roll salmon inside the mixture so it coats salmon all over.
3. Serve with green leafy salad.

# Coq Au Vin

## INGREDIENTS (FOR 8 SERVINGS)

- 3 tbsp. of fresh parsley (chopped)
- 1 bouquet garni
- 450 g of button mushrooms
- 2 tbsp. of plain flour
- 100 g of streaky bacon (chopped)
- 2 red onions (chopped)
- 2 tbsp. of olive oil
- 16 chicken thighs (skin removed)
- 3 carrots (chopped)
- 3 cloves of garlic (crushed)

## COOKING DIRECTIONS

1. Pre-heat oven to 180C/360F.
2. Pour the flour in a large flat tray.
3. Roll the chicken in the tray so the flour coats the chicken.
4. Place large saucepan over heat and add olive oil to heat up.
5. Add chicken to the pan and brown on all sides.
6. Remove chickens and set aside.
7. Add bacon to the pan and fry. Remove and set aside.
8. Add onions to the pan and sauté for 5 minutes.
9. Add red wine and stir. Scrape the bottom and sides of the pan to free up any residue.
10. Add the chickens and garlic, carrots and bouquet garni. Stir.
11. Pour everything into a large ovenproof dish.
12. Bake for 1 hour.
13. Remove dish from oven and remove any excess fat and the bouquet garni.
14. Add mushrooms and return the dish to the oven.
15. Let it bake for another 15 minutes.
16. Remove from the oven, stir in parsley.
17. Serve.

# Turkey Satay Skewers

## INGREDIENTS (FOR 4 SERVINGS)

- 2 tsp. of soy sauce
- 250 g turkey breast (cubed
- 200 ml of coconut milk
- 25 g of smooth peanut butter
- 1/2 tsp. of ground turmeric
- 1/2 of a Bird's eye chili (finely chopped)
- 1 clove of garlic (crushed)

## COOKING DIRECTIONS

1. Pour coconut milk in a mixing bowl. Add turmeric, peanut butter, chili, garlic and soy sauce. Mix.
2. Add turkey to the mixing bowl and stir so the mixture coats the turkey all over.
3. Thread turkey onto skewers.
4. Grill for 5 minutes, flip and grill the other side for another 5 minutes
5. Serve.

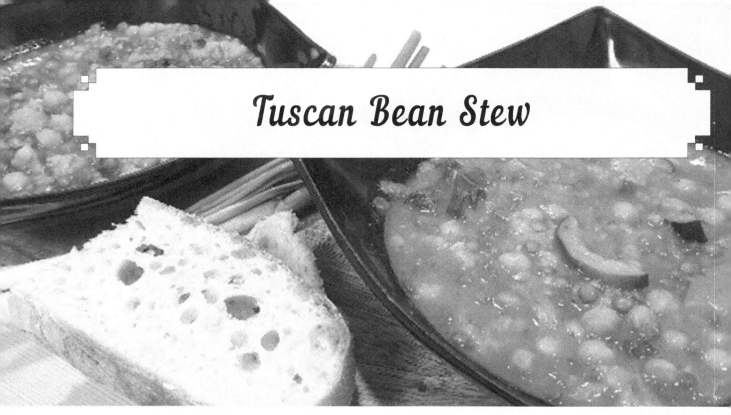

# Tuscan Bean Stew

## INGREDIENTS (FOR 2 SERVINGS)

- 40 g buckwheat
- 50 g red onion (finely chopped)
- 50 g kale (roughly chopped)
- 30 g carrot (peeled and finely chopped)
- 200 g canned mixed beans
- 30 g celery (trimmed and finely chopped)
- 1 tsp. of tomato purée
- 1 garlic clove (finely chopped)
- 1400 g canned chopped Italian tomatoes
- 1/2 Bird's eye chili (finely chopped)
- 200 ml vegetable stock
- 1 tsp. of herbs de Provence

## COOKING DIRECTIONS

1. Cook buckwheat according to the instructions on the package. Set aside and keep warm.
2. Place a medium-sized saucepan over heat and add oil to heat up.
3. Add onions, garlic, carrot, chili, celery, herbs and stir-fry until onions are soft.
4. Add tomato puree and stock tomatoes and stir. Bring to a boil.
5. Add beans and let it simmer for 30 minutes.
6. Add kale and continue to cook for another 7 minutes.
7. Add parsley and stir.
8. Serve stew with cooked buckwheat.

# Chinese-style Pork with Pak Choi

## INGREDIENTS (FOR 4 SERVINGS)

- 400 g pork mince
- 400 g firm tofu, cut into large cubes
- 100 g beansprouts
- 20 g parsley, chopped
- 200g pak choi
- 100 g shiitake mushrooms, sliced
- 1 tbsp. of corn flour
- a 5cm fresh ginger root (peeled and grated)
- 1 tbsp. of water
- 1 tbsp. of rapeseed oil
- 1 shallot (peeled and sliced)
- 125 ml chicken stock
- 1 clove garlic (peeled and crushed)
- 1 tbsp. of rice wine
- 1 tbsp. of soy sauce
- 1 tsp. of brown sugar
- 1 tbsp. of tomato paste

## COOKING DIRECTIONS

1. Spread kitchen towels on a tray and place your tofu on the towels.
2. Cover it up with another set of kitchen towels.
3. In a large mixing bowl, mix water and corn flour, making sure no lumps remain.
4. Add rice wine, chicken stock, brown sugar, tomato puree, soy sauce, ginger and crushed garlic. Mix everything together.
5. Place a frying pan over high heat and add oil to heat up.
6. Stir-fry shiitake mushrooms in the pan for 3 minutes. Use a slotted spoon to remove the mushrooms and set aside.
7. Add tofu to the pan and stir-fry until golden brown on all sides.
8. Add pak choi and shallots to the pan and continue to stir-fry for another 2 minutes.
9. Add pork mince and continue to stir-fry until the pork is cooked through.
10. Now, reduce the heat and add the sauce.
11. Add the shiitake mushrooms back to the pan and stir.
12. Add beansprouts and stir.
13. Cook for 3 minutes and remove from heat.
14. Add parsley and stir.
15. Serve.

# Snacks And Dessert Recipes

# Honey Chili Nuts

## INGREDIENTS (FOR 20 SERVINGS)

- 1/2 Bird's eye chili (deseeded and finely chopped)
- 150 g of walnuts
- 1 tbsp. of honey
- 150 g of pecan nuts
- 50 g of softened butter

## COOKING DIRECTIONS

1. Preheat your oven to 170C/325F.
2. Add all ingredients to a bowl and mix.
3. Spread on a baking sheet lined with parchment paper and bake for 10 minutes.
4. Remove from oven, allow it cool up, and serve.

# Raw Brownie Bites

## INGREDIENTS (FOR 6 SERVINGS)

- 1 cup of cacao powder
- 2 1/2 cups of whole walnuts
- 1/4 tsp. of sea salt
- 1/4 cup of almonds
- 1 tsp. of vanilla extract
- 2 1/2 cups of Medjool dates

## COOKING DIRECTIONS

1. Add all your ingredients to a food processor and process until well combined
2. Roll the mixture into balls and place each ball on your baking sheet.
3. Place in the refrigerator for 2 hours.
4. Enjoy.

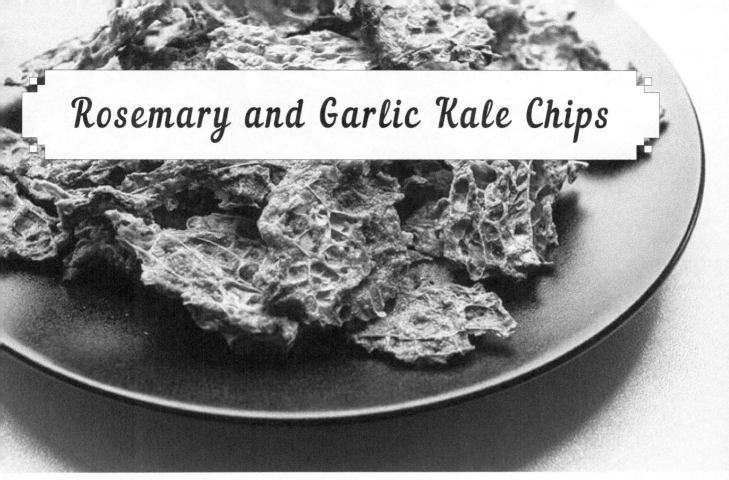

# Rosemary and Garlic Kale Chips

## INGREDIENTS (FOR 6 SERVINGS)

- 2 tbsp. of olive oil
- 250 g kale chips (chopped)
- 2 cloves of garlic

- 2 sprigs of rosemary
- Sea salt and freshly ground black pepper to taste

## COOKING DIRECTIONS

1. Preheat your oven to 170C/325F.
2. Place a saucepan over low heat and add olive oil to heat up.
3. Add rosemary and garlic, sauté for 10 minutes.
4. Remove garlic and rosemary from the oil and discard it.
5. Now add kale leaves to the infused oil and toss to coat.
6. Season coated kale leaves with salt and pepper.
7. Spread kale on 2 baking sheets.
8. Bake in the oven for 15 minutes.
9. Serve.

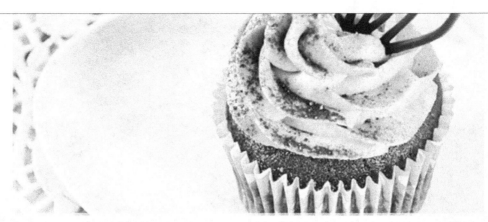

# Chocolate Cupcakes with Matcha Icing

## INGREDIENTS (FOR 12 SERVINGS)

For Cupcakes:
- 120 ml boiling water
- 120 ml milk
- 50 ml vegetable oil
- 60 g cocoa
- 200 g caster sugar
- 150 g self-rising flour
- 1 egg
- 1/2 tsp. of vanilla extract
- 1/2 tsp. of fine espresso coffee (or decaf)
- 1/2 tsp. salt

For Icing:
- 50 g of soft cream cheese
- 50 g of butter (room temperature)
- 1/2 tsp. of vanilla bean paste
- 1 tbsp. of Matcha green tea powder
- 50 g of icing sugar

## COOKING DIRECTIONS

1. Pre-heat your oven to 180C/360F.
2. Line 12 cupcake tins with parchment paper.
3. Combine espresso powder, flour, salt, sugar, and cocoa in a large mixing bowl. Mix together.
4. In another bowl, mix vegetable oil, milk, vanilla extract and egg together.
5. Pour the egg mixture into the flour mixture and use a hand-held electric mixer to mix everything together until well combined.
6. Start adding the boiling water slowly and continue to use the electric mixer to beat it on low speed. The batter is going to be a bit more watery than your regular cake batter.
7. When you finish adding the water, beat it on high speed for 1 more minutes to air the batter.
8. Spoon the batter into your cupcake tins.
9. Bake in the oven for 15 to 20 minutes.
10. While the cake is baking, make your icing cream. Just combine the icing sugar with butter and mix until smooth. Then add Matcha powder and vanilla and continue to beat it until everything is well Incorporated.
11. Lastly add cream cheese and mix until smooth and Incorporated.
12. Serve the icing over the cakes.

# Pizza Kale Chips

## INGREDIENTS (FOR 6 SERVINGS)

- 100 ml of water
- 250 g of kale (chopped into 2-inch pieces)
- 2 tbsp. of olive oil
- 50 g of ground almonds

- 1/2 tsp. of onion powder
- 50 g of Parmesan cheese
- 1/2 tsp. of oregano
- 3 tbsp. of tomato puree
- 1/2 tsp. of mixed herbs

## COOKING DIRECTIONS

1. Preheat your oven to 170C/325F.
2. Add all ingredients except kale to a food processor and process until as smooth as can be.
3. Pour the mixture in a bowl and toss chopped kale in it so it can coat the kale.
4. Spread kale on 2 baking sheets.
5. Bake in the oven for 15 minutes.
6. Serve.

# Choc Nut Truffles

## INGREDIENTS (FOR 8 SERVINGS)

- 1 tbsp. of coconut oil
- 150 g of shredded coconut
- 2 tbsp. of cocoa powder
- 4 Medjool dates
- 25 g hazelnuts (chopped)
- 50 g walnuts

## COOKING DIRECTIONS

1. Add all ingredients to a food processor and process until it becomes a smooth paste.
2. Use a teaspoon to scoop the paste and roll each spoonful into a ball.
3. Arrange the balls on a tray lined with foil paper.
4. Let it sit in the refrigerator for an hour.
5. Serve.

# Sirtfood Hummus with Celery

## INGREDIENTS (FOR 4 SERVINGS)

- 1 tbsp. of olive oil
- Juice of 1 lemon
- 8 sticks of celery (cut into batons)
- 1 tbsp. of tahini

- 175 g chickpeas
- 1 tbsp. of fresh parsley (chopped)
- 2 cloves of garlic (crushed)

## COOKING DIRECTIONS

1. Add garlic, chickpeas, lemon juice, tahini paste, to a blender and process until smooth and creamy.
2. Transfer to serving bowls and serve with celery sticks on the sides.

# Strawberry Flapjacks

## INGREDIENTS (FOR 8 SERVINGS)

- 2 tbsp. of 100% cocoa powder
- 75 g of porridge oats
- 1 tbsp. of coconut oil
- 125 g of dates
- 50 g of walnuts
- 50 g of strawberries
- 50 g of unsalted peanuts

## COOKING DIRECTIONS

1. Add all ingredients to a food processor and process until it becomes a smooth, thick paste.
2. Pour the paste on a baking sheet with foil paper.
3. Use your hands to press it down and smoothen it.
4. Use a cookie cutter to cut it into 8 pieces.
5. Sprinkle cocoa powder all over it.

# Spicy Poached Apples

## INGREDIENTS (FOR 4 SERVINGS)

- 300 ml of green tea
- 4 apples
- 2 cinnamon sticks
- 4 star anise
- 2 tbsp. of honey

## COOKING DIRECTIONS

1. Place a saucepan over heat and add green tea and honey. Stir and bring to a boil.
2. Add cinnamon, star anise and apples. Stir for 15 minutes.
3. Serve.

# Chocolate Balls

## INGREDIENTS (FOR 6 SERVINGS)

- 1 tbsp. of cocoa powder
- 50 g of peanut butter
- 1 tbsp. of honey

- 25 g of shredded coconut
- 25 g of cocoa powder

## COOKING DIRECTIONS

1. Add all ingredients to a bowl and mix well.
2. Use a tsp. to scoop the paste and roll each spoonful into a ball.
3. Arrange the balls on a tray lined with foil paper.
4. Let it sit in the refrigerator for an hour.
5. Serve.

# Pistachio Fudge

## INGREDIENTS (FOR 10 SERVINGS)

- 2 tbsp. of water
- 225 g Medjool dates
- 25 g of oats
- 50 g of desiccated coconuts
- 100 g of pistachio nuts (shelled)

## COOKING DIRECTIONS

1. Add all ingredients to a food processor and process until it becomes a smooth paste.
2. Spread the mixture on a tray lined with foil paper. Cut into 10 pieces.
3. Let it sit in the refrigerator for an hour.
4. Serve.

# *Warm Berries Cream*

## INGREDIENTS (FOR 4 SERVINGS)

- Juice of 1 orange
- Zest of 1 orange
- 4 tbsp. of fresh whipped cream
- 100 g of blackberries
- 100 g of redcurrants
- 250 g of strawberries
- 250 g of blueberries

## COOKING DIRECTIONS

1. Place a small pan over heat and add orange juice, honey and berries. Let it simmer for 5 minutes.
2. Serve with a dollop of whipped cream.

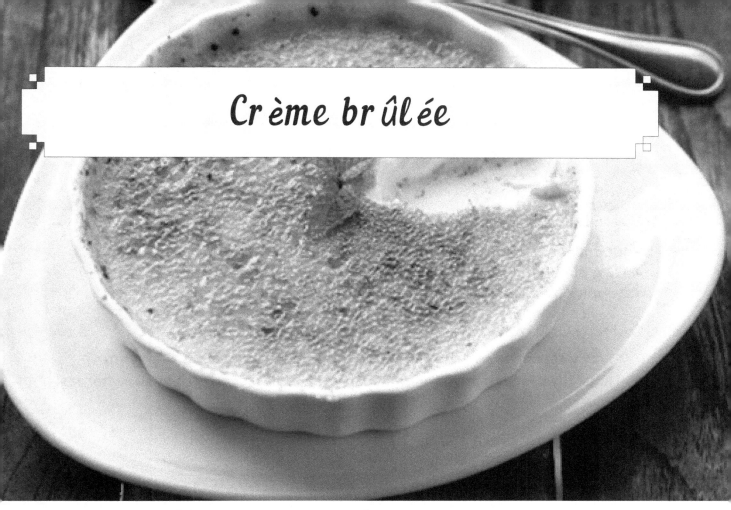

# Crème brûlée

## INGREDIENTS (FOR 4 SERVINGS)

- 400 g of strawberries
- 100 g of brown sugar
- 1 tsp. of vanilla extract
- 125 g Greek yogurt
- 300 g plain low-fat yogurt

## COOKING DIRECTIONS

1. Divide the strawberries among 4 ramekins.
2. Mix vanilla extract and plain yogurt together and pour it over the strawberries in the ramekins.
3. Add a scoop of Greek yogurt on top.
4. Add a sprinkle of brown sugar on top.
5. Place ramekins on a grill and grill for 4 minutes.
6. Serve.

# Chocolate Fondue

## INGREDIENTS (FOR 4 SERVINGS)

- 100 ml heavy cream
- 125 g of dark 85% chocolate
- 2 apples (peeled, cored and sliced)
- 200 g cherries
- 300 g strawberries

## COOKING DIRECTIONS

1. Place a saucepan over heat and add cream and chocolate. Let it warm up.
2. Transfer to serving bowls and garnish with apples, cherries and strawberries.

# Chocolate Brownies

## INGREDIENTS (FOR 14 SERVINGS)

- 1/2 tsp. of baking soda
- 200 g of 85% dark chocolate
- 2 tsp. of vanilla essence
- 100 g of walnuts (chopped)
- 25 ml coconut oil (melted)
- 3 eggs

## COOKING DIRECTIONS

1. Pre-heat your oven to 180C/350F.
2. Add eggs, dates, coconut oil, chocolate, vanilla, and baking soda to a food processor and process until smooth.
3. Add walnuts and stir.
4. Pour everything inside a baking tray and bake for 30 minutes.
5. Cut into smaller pieces and serve.

# Frozen Strawberry Yoghurt

## INGREDIENTS (FOR 4 SERVINGS)

- 1 tbsp. of honey
- 450 g of plain yogurt
- Juice of 1 orange
- 175 g of strawberries

## COOKING DIRECTIONS

1. Add orange juice and strawberries to a food processor and process until smooth.
2. Sieve to remove the seeds.
3. Add yogurt and honey and stir.
4. Let it sit in your refrigerator for an hour.
5. Serve.

# Raspberry and Blackcurrant Jelly

## INGREDIENTS (FOR 2 SERVINGS)

- 100 g blackcurrant (washed and stalks removed)
- 100 g raspberries (washed)
- 300 ml water
- 2 tbsp. of granulated sugar
- 2 leaves of gelatin

## COOKING DIRECTIONS

1. Place gelatin leaves in cold water to soften.
2. Place a small saucepan over heat and add sugar and 100ml of water. Bring to a boil.
3. Let it simmer for 5 minutes.
4. Remove from heat and let it cool down for 2 minutes.
5. Remove gelatin leaves from water and squeeze out excess water.
6. Add gelatin leaves to the pan and stir continuously until it completely dissolves.
7. Add the remaining water.
8. Arrange raspberries in serving dishes.
9. Pour the jelly on top of the raspberries in the serving dishes.
10. Refrigerate for 4 hours.
11. Enjoy.

# Sirtfood Bites

## INGREDIENTS (FOR 4 SERVINGS)

- 250 g Medjool dates, pitted
- 30 g dark chocolate (85% cocoa solids, broken into pieces)
- 120 g walnuts
- 2 tbsp. of water
- 1 tsp. of vanilla extract
- 1 tbsp. of Extra virgin olive oil
- 1 tbsp. of cocoa powder
- 1 tbsp. of ground turmeric

## COOKING DIRECTIONS

1. Pour chocolate and walnuts in your food processor and process until it turns into powder.
2. Add everything else (except water) to the blender and process into a smooth mixture.
3. Add water in bits to make it into a thick paste and roll it into bite-sized balls.
4. Refrigerate for a few hours.
5. Serve.

# Dressings And Sauce Recipes

# Teriyaki Sauce

## INGREDIENTS (FOR 4 SERVINGS)

- 1 tsp. of red wine vinegar
- 2 cloves of garlic
- 200 ml soy sauce
- 1 inch of fresh ginger root (peeled and grated)
- 200 ml pineapple juice

## COOKING DIRECTIONS

1. Place a saucepan on the stove and add all the ingredients.
2. Stir and bring to a boil.
3. Allow it to cool up.
4. Discard garlic and ginger.
5. Serve with tofu dishes or use as marinade for meat or fish.

# Basil and Walnut Pesto Dressing

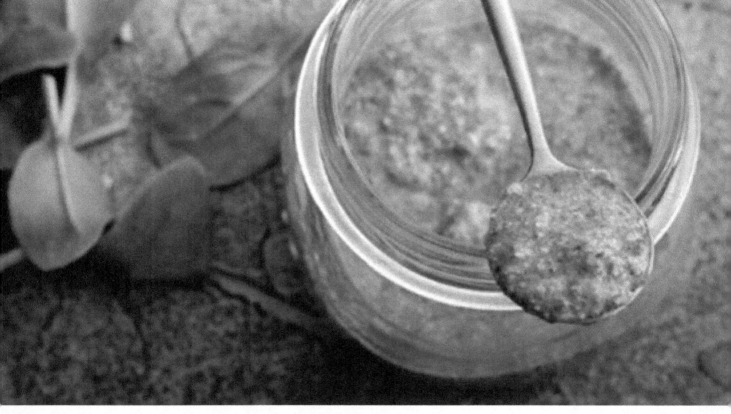

## INGREDIENTS (FOR 2 SERVINGS)

- 25 g of walnuts
- 4 tbsp. of olive oil
- 50 g of fresh basil

- 2 tbsp. of Parmesan cheese (grated)
- 3 cloves of garlic (crushed)
- 50 g of walnuts

## COOKING DIRECTIONS

1. Combine all ingredients into your blender or food processor, and blend until smooth.
2. Preserve in your refrigerator and serve with pasta, salads, meat or fish.

# Lemon Caper Pesto Dressing

## INGREDIENTS (FOR 8 SERVINGS)

- 1 tbsp. of lemon juice
- 6 tbsp. of fresh parsley leaves
- 2 tbsp. of olive oil
- 50 g of cashew nuts
- 2 tbsp. of capers
- 3 cloves of garlic

## COOKING DIRECTIONS

1. Combine all ingredients into your blender or food processor, and blend until smooth.
2. Preserve in your refrigerator and serve with pasta, salads, meat or fish.

# Turmeric and Lemon Dressing

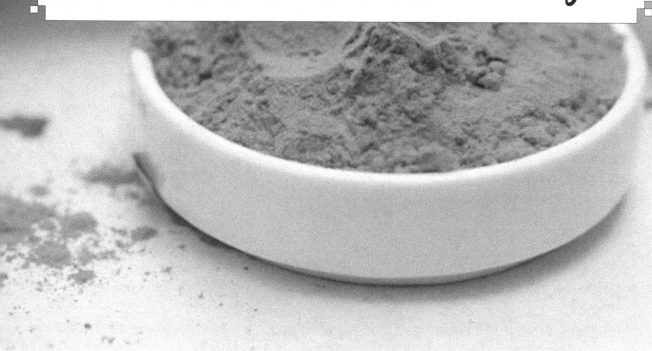

## INGREDIENTS (FOR 4 SERVINGS)

- Juice of 1 lemon
- 4 tbsp. of olive oil
- 1 tsp. of turmeric

## COOKING DIRECTIONS

1. Put all the ingredients in a mason jar and shake to combine.
2. Serve over salad.

# Parsley Pesto Dressing

## INGREDIENTS (FOR 8 SERVINGS)

- 6 tbsp. of fresh parsley leaves
- 2 tbsp. of olive oil
- 2 cloves of garlic
- 75 g of Parmesan cheese (finely grated)
- 50 g of pine nuts

## COOKING DIRECTIONS

1. Combine all ingredients into your blender or food processor, and blend until smooth.
2. Preserve in your refrigerator and serve with pasta, salads, meat or fish.

# Garlic Vinaigrette Dressing

## INGREDIENTS (FOR 4 SERVINGS)

- Freshly ground black pepper to taste
- 1 clove of garlic (crushed)
- 1 tbsp. of lemon juice
- 4 tbsp. of olive oil

## COOKING DIRECTIONS

1. Put all the ingredients in a mason jar and shake to combine.
2. Serve over salad.

# Walnut and Mint Pesto Dressing

## INGREDIENTS (FOR 8 SERVINGS)

- 1 tbsp. of lemon juice
- 6 tbsp. of fresh mint leaves
- 100 g of Parmesan cheese
- 2 cloves of garlic
- 50 g of walnuts

## COOKING DIRECTIONS

1. Combine all ingredients into your blender or food processor, and blend until smooth.
2. Preserve in your refrigerator and serve with pasta, salads, meat or fish.

# Walnut Vinaigrette Dressing

## INGREDIENTS (FOR 8 SERVINGS)

- 6 tbsp. of olive oil
- 1 clove of garlic (finely chopped)
- 1 tbsp. of walnut oil
- 3 tbsp. of red wine vinegar
- Sea salt and freshly ground black pepper to taste

## COOKING DIRECTIONS

1. Put all the ingredients in a mason jar and shake to combine.
2. Serve over salad.

Your feedback is very important to us, it gives us the support and power to bring our best recipes into your kitchen for you and your families.

Do not forget to leave a review honest. We appreciate it very much.

Thanks

## Customer Reviews

☆☆☆☆☆ 15

5.0 out of 5 stars ▾

| | | |
|---|---|---|
| 5 star | | 100% |
| 4 star | | 0% |
| 3 star | | 0% |
| 2 star | | 0% |
| 1 star | | 0% |

Share your thoughts with other customers

Write a customer review

CPSIA information can be obtained
at www.ICGtesting.com
Printed in the USA
BVHW061021071220
595088BV00005B/243